Reversing Heart Valve Disease

*The Complete Guide to Understanding
Cardiovascular Issues, Finding the Best
Treatment Options, and Reclaiming Your Health*

| Things You Must Know |

Isabella White

Copyright © 2023 by Isabella White

Disclaimer: The information provided in this book has not been evaluated by the FDA and is not intended to diagnose, treat, cure, or prevent any disease or health condition. The content is for informational and educational purposes only. It is not meant as a substitute for medical advice from your physician or other medical professional. Please consult a qualified health provider for any health concerns. The author and publisher disclaim any responsibility for any adverse effects from applying the information provided herein.

About the Book

A diagnosis of heart valve disease can make you feel worried and uncertain about the future. As a patient, you likely have many questions about what is happening inside your heart and your options. In this book, writer and nurse Isabella White uses her 15 years of experience working with heart valve patients to provide clear, supportive information to guide you through this challenging time.

Isabella explains the basics of how heart valves work in simple terms, the types of valve problems, and the range of symptoms they may cause. She describes the surgical and less-invasive treatments available and offers down-to-earth advice on choosing the right approach for your unique situation. Isabella provides practical tips on getting ready for surgery, managing discomfort during recovery, safely returning to normal activities, adopting a healthy lifestyle, and controlling heart health.

Isabella understands the emotional impact heart valve disease can have. She shares suggestions on building a support network, setting realistic goals, and keeping an upbeat frame of mind—all key ingredients for healing.

Suppose you or a loved one has been diagnosed with a heart valve issue. This book provides the knowledge, insights, and encouragement to recover, reverse damage, and reclaim health.

Table of Contents

About the Book_____ 2

Introduction_____ 6

Chapter 1
Understanding Heart Valve Disease_____ 8

Anatomy and Function of Heart Valves_____ 8

Types of Valve Problems and Diseases_____ 12

Symptoms and Complications_____17

Diagnosis and Testing_____23

Chapter 2
Treatment Options for Faulty Heart Valves___27

Medications for Managing Symptoms_____ 27

Open-Heart Surgery for Valve Repair and
Replacement_____30

Minimally Invasive Transcatheter Procedures_33

Choosing the Right Treatment Approach_____ 38

Chapter 3
Preparing for Heart Valve Surgery_____ 42

Finding the Right Cardiac Surgeon_____ 42

What to Expect Before, During, and
After Surgery_____45

Recovery Process and Rehabilitation_____49

Chapter 4

Life After Heart Valve Surgery_____ 56

    Follow-Up Care and Monitoring_____56

    Managing Pain and Discomfort_____ 62

    Returning to Normal Activities_____69

    Diet and Lifestyle Guidelines_____ 76

Chapter 5

Improving Your Cardiovascular Health_____ 86

    Managing Heart Disease Risk Factors_____ 86

    Nutrition and Exercise for Heart Health_____ 99

    Stress and Management Techniques_____ 105

    Supplements and Alternative Therapies_____ 111

Chapter 6

Living Well with Heart Valve Disease_____ 123

    Setting Goals and Milestones_____ 123

    Travel and Leisure Considerations_____127

    Long-Term Outlook_____ 130

Conclusion_____ 133

Appendix_____ 137

    Glossary_____ 138

    References_____142

Introduction

If you've been diagnosed with heart valve disease, it's understandable to feel worried and have many questions. What exactly is wrong with your heart? What will treatment involve? Will you be able to get back to a normal life? This book was written to provide clear, practical answers and information during this challenging time.

As a medical writer and nurse with 15 years of experience working directly with heart valve patients, I've seen firsthand the physical and emotional impact this diagnosis can have. I aim to help educate and empower you to participate actively in your care. Knowledge is power when it comes to managing heart health.

In the following chapters, I explain how healthy heart valves work, the types of valve diseases, and the symptoms they can cause. I describe your treatment options in plain terms, including medications, surgery, and less invasive procedures.

You'll learn practical tips on preparing for any procedures, setting reasonable expectations for recovery, sticking to lifestyle changes, and taking control of your cardiovascular health. I also offer suggestions for coping with the emotional side of this diagnosis, like creating a support network, managing stress, and maintaining motivation.

It is possible to reverse the damage, recover fully, and reclaim your life after a heart valve diagnosis. The information in this book will help make your journey a story of healing, health, and new beginnings.

Chapter 1

Understanding Heart Valve Disease

Anatomy and Function of Heart Valves

The heart is a muscular organ that pumps blood throughout the body. Blood carries oxygen and nutrients to cells and tissues, removing carbon dioxide and waste products. The heart has four valves that act like gates to ensure blood flows in the right direction and pressure. These valves are:

- The tricuspid valve, which separates the right atrium (upper chamber) and the right ventricle (lower chamber) of the heart.

- The pulmonary valve, which separates the right ventricle, and the pulmonary artery, which carries blood to the lungs.

- The mitral valve, which separates the left atrium and left ventricle of the heart.
- The aortic valve, which separates the left ventricle, and the aorta, which carries blood to the rest of the body.

Each valve has two or three flaps of tissue, called leaflets or cusps, that open and close to allow blood to pass through. The valves are attached to the heart's inner wall by thin cords of tissue called chordae tendineae, which prevent the valves from flipping inside out. The valves are also supported by muscles in the heart wall, called papillary muscles, which contract and relax to help the valves open and close.

The valves work in coordination with the contraction and relaxation of the heart chambers. When the atria contract, they push blood into the ventricles through the tricuspid and mitral valves. When the ventricles contract, they push blood into the pulmonary artery and the aorta through the pulmonary and aortic valves. When the chambers relax, the valves close to prevent blood from flowing back into the heart.

The opening and closing of the valves produce the sound of the heartbeat, which can be heard with a stethoscope. The first heart sound (S1) is caused by the closure of the tricuspid and mitral valves at the beginning of ventricular contraction. The second heart sound (S2) is caused by the closure of the pulmonary and aortic valves at the end of ventricular contraction. Sometimes, a third (S3) or fourth (S4) heart sound can be heard, which may indicate abnormal heart function.

The normal function of the heart valves is essential for maintaining adequate blood flow and pressure throughout the body. If the valves become damaged or diseased, they may not open or close properly, causing blood to leak or flow backward. This can reduce the amount of blood that reaches the organs and tissues and increase the heart's workload. Some common causes and types of heart valve disease are:

- Congenital heart defects, which are present at birth and affect the structure or development of the heart valves.

- Rheumatic fever, which is an inflammatory condition that can result from untreated strep throat and damage the heart valves.
- Infective endocarditis, which is an infection of the heart's inner lining or the heart valves, is usually caused by bacteria or fungi.
- Degenerative valve disease, which is the wear and tear of the heart valves due to aging or other factors.
- Calcific aortic stenosis, which is the narrowing of the aortic valve due to calcium deposits on the leaflets.
- Mitral valve prolapse, which is the bulging of one or both leaflets of the mitral valve into the left atrium during ventricular contraction.
- Mitral valve regurgitation, which is the leakage of blood from the left ventricle to the left atrium through the mitral valve.
- Aortic valve regurgitation, which is the blood leakage from the aorta to the left ventricle through the aortic valve.

Heart valve disease can cause various symptoms, such as chest pain, shortness of breath, fatigue, dizziness, palpitations, swelling of the legs or abdomen, and fainting.

Types of Valve Problems and Diseases

Heart valve problems and diseases affect the normal function of one or more of the four heart valves: the aortic, mitral, pulmonary, and tricuspid valves. These valves regulate the flow and direction of blood through the heart and to the rest of the body. When the valves become damaged or diseased, they can cause various symptoms and complications that can affect the quality of life and even be life-threatening.

There are two main heart valve problems and diseases: stenosis and regurgitation. Stenosis is the narrowing or stiffening of the valve opening, which reduces the amount of blood that can flow through the valve. Regurgitation is the leakage or backflow of blood through the valve, which prevents the valve from closing completely. Both stenosis and regurgitation can cause the heart to work harder to pump blood, which can lead to heart failure, arrhythmias, and other problems.

Stenosis and regurgitation can affect any of the four heart valves, but some valves are more prone to certain problems than others. The most common types of heart valve problems and diseases are:

- **Aortic stenosis.** This is the narrowing of the aortic valve, which separates the left ventricle and the aorta. Aortic stenosis can be caused by congenital disabilities, such as a bicuspid aortic valve, or by degenerative changes, such as calcification or scarring, due to aging or other factors. Aortic stenosis can cause symptoms such as chest pain, shortness of breath, fatigue, dizziness, and fainting. Aortic stenosis can also increase the risk of stroke, heart attack, and sudden cardiac death.

- **Aortic regurgitation.** This is the leakage of blood from the aorta back into the left ventricle through the aortic valve. Congenital disabilities, such as a bicuspid aortic valve, or acquired conditions, such as infective endocarditis, rheumatic fever, trauma, or aortic dissection, can cause aortic regurgitation. Aortic regurgitation can cause symptoms such as palpitations, shortness of breath, swelling of the legs or abdomen, and fatigue. Aortic regurgitation can also lead to heart failure, arrhythmias, and endocarditis.

- **Mitral stenosis.** This is the narrowing of the mitral valve, which separates the left atrium and the left ventricle. Mitral stenosis is usually caused by rheumatic fever, which is an inflammatory condition that can result from untreated strep throat. Mitral stenosis can cause symptoms such as shortness of breath, coughing, fatigue, swelling of the legs or abdomen, and chest pain. Mitral stenosis can also increase the risk of atrial fibrillation, stroke, pulmonary hypertension, and infection.

- **Mitral regurgitation.** This is the leakage of blood from the left ventricle back into the left atrium through the mitral valve. Congenital disabilities, such as a cleft mitral valve, or by acquired conditions, such as mitral valve prolapse, infective endocarditis, rheumatic fever, cardiomyopathy, or ischemic heart disease, can cause mitral regurgitation. Mitral regurgitation can cause symptoms such as shortness of breath, fatigue, palpitations, and chest pain. Mitral regurgitation can also lead to heart failure, arrhythmias, and endocarditis.

- **Pulmonary stenosis.** This is the narrowing of the pulmonary valve, which separates the right ventricle and the pulmonary artery. Pulmonary stenosis is usually a congenital disability that affects the development of the valve. Pulmonary stenosis can cause cyanosis (bluish skin color), shortness of breath, fatigue, and chest pain. Pulmonary stenosis can also affect the growth and development of the heart and lungs.

- **Pulmonary regurgitation.** This is the leakage of blood from the pulmonary artery back into the right ventricle through the pulmonary valve. Pulmonary regurgitation is usually a complication of pulmonary hypertension, which is high blood pressure in the lungs. Pulmonary regurgitation can cause symptoms such as shortness of breath, fatigue, swelling of the legs or abdomen, and chest pain. Pulmonary regurgitation can also lead to right-sided heart failure and arrhythmias.

- **Tricuspid stenosis.** This narrows the tricuspid valve, which separates the right atrium and ventricle. Tricuspid stenosis is rare and is usually caused by rheumatic fever or infective endocarditis. Tricuspid stenosis can cause symptoms such as fatigue, swelling of the legs or abdomen, and abdominal pain. Tricuspid stenosis can also increase the risk of atrial fibrillation, infection, and liver problems.

- **Tricuspid regurgitation.** This is the leakage of blood from the right ventricle back into the right atrium through the tricuspid valve. Tricuspid regurgitation can be caused by congenital disabilities, such as Ebstein's anomaly, or by acquired conditions, such as pulmonary hypertension, infective endocarditis, rheumatic fever, or right-sided heart failure. Tricuspid regurgitation can cause symptoms such as fatigue, swelling of the legs or abdomen, and abdominal pain.

Tricuspid regurgitation can also worsen the symptoms and complications of pulmonary hypertension and right-sided heart failure.

Symptoms and Complications

Heart valve disease can affect people's quality of life and health. Different symptoms and complications may occur depending on the type and severity of the valve problem. Some of the common symptoms and complications of heart valve disease are:

- **Shortness of breath.** This is the feeling of not being able to breathe enough or comfortably. It can occur at rest, during physical activity, or when lying down or bending over. It can be caused by reduced blood flow to the lungs, increased pressure, or fluid buildup in the lungs due to heart failure.
- **Fatigue.** This is the feeling of being tired, weak, or exhausted. It can occur due to reduced blood flow to the body, increased workload of the heart, or anemia (low red blood cell count).

- **Chest pain.** This is the feeling of discomfort, pressure, or squeezing in the chest. It can occur due to reduced blood flow to the heart muscle, increased pressure in the heart chambers, or inflammation of the heart lining. Chest pain can be a sign of angina (chest pain due to coronary artery disease) or a heart attack.

- **Dizziness.** This is the feeling of being lightheaded, faint, or unsteady. It can occur due to reduced blood flow to the brain, low blood pressure, or abnormal heart rhythms. Dizziness can lead to fainting (loss of consciousness) or falls.

- **Palpitations.** This is the feeling of having a fast, irregular, or skipped heartbeat. It can occur due to abnormal electrical signals in the heart, increased pressure in the heart chambers, or valve leakage or narrowing. Palpitations can cause anxiety, discomfort, or chest pain.

- **Swelling.** This is the tissue's fluid buildup, especially in the legs, feet, or abdomen. It can occur due to reduced blood flow from the heart, increased pressure in the veins, or fluid retention due to heart failure. Swelling can cause pain, discomfort, or difficulty moving.

- **Stroke.** This is a sudden interruption of blood flow to the brain, causing brain damage. It can occur due to a blood clot or a bleeding vessel in the brain. Stroke can be caused by valve disease in several ways, such as:

  o A blood clot can form on a damaged or infected valve and travel to the brain, blocking a blood vessel. This is called an embolic stroke.

  o A blood clot can form in the heart due to atrial fibrillation, a common arrhythmia associated with valve disease, and travel to the brain, blocking a blood vessel. This is also called an embolic stroke.

  o A narrowed or leaky valve can reduce the blood flow and pressure to the brain, causing a lack of oxygen and nutrients. This is called an ischemic stroke.

> ○ A leaky valve can increase the blood pressure in the brain, causing a blood vessel to rupture and bleed. This is called a hemorrhagic stroke.

Stroke can cause symptoms such as sudden weakness, numbness, or paralysis of the face, arm, or leg, especially on one side of the body; sudden confusion; trouble speaking or understanding; sudden vision problems; sudden dizziness; loss of balance; difficulty walking; or a sudden severe headache. A stroke is a medical emergency that requires immediate treatment to prevent permanent disability or death.

- **Heart failure.** This is a condition in which the heart cannot pump enough blood to meet the body's needs. It can occur due to valve disease in several ways, such as:
  - ○ A narrowed or leaky valve can reduce the blood flow out of the heart, causing the heart to work harder and become enlarged and weakened over time. This is called systolic heart failure.

- ○ A leaky valve can increase the blood pressure and volume in the heart, causing the heart to become stiff and unable to relax and fill properly. This is called diastolic heart failure.
- ○ A leaky valve can cause blood to go back into the lungs or the body, causing fluid buildup and congestion. This is called congestive heart failure.

Heart failure can cause symptoms such as shortness of breath, fatigue, swelling, coughing, weight gain, loss of appetite, nausea, or abdominal pain. Heart failure can also lead to complications such as kidney damage, liver damage, or arrhythmias. Heart failure is a chronic and progressive condition that requires lifelong management and treatment.

- **Endocarditis.** This is an infection of the inner lining of the heart or the heart valves, usually caused by bacteria or fungi. It can occur due to valve disease in several ways, such as:
  - ○ A damaged or diseased valve can provide a site for bacteria or fungi to

attach and grow, forming a mass of infected tissue called vegetation. This can damage the valve further and cause regurgitation or stenosis.

- o Vegetation can break off and travel through the bloodstream, causing infections in other body parts, such as the brain, lungs, kidneys, or skin. This can also cause embolic strokes or abscesses.
- o An infection can spread from the valve to the heart muscle, causing inflammation and damage. This can lead to heart failure or arrhythmias.

Endocarditis can cause symptoms such as fever, chills, night sweats, weight loss, fatigue, joint or muscle pain, or a new or changed heart murmur. Endocarditis can be life-threatening and requires prompt diagnosis and treatment with antibiotics and sometimes surgery.

Diagnosis and Testing

To diagnose heart valve disease, your doctor will ask about your medical history, symptoms, and family history of heart problems. Your doctor will also perform a physical exam, which may include listening to your heart with a stethoscope, checking your pulse and blood pressure, and looking for signs of fluid buildup in your body.

Your doctor may order one or more tests to confirm the diagnosis of heart valve disease and to assess the type, severity, and impact of the valve problem on your heart and body. Some of the common tests for heart valve disease are:

- **Echocardiogram.** This is the main test for diagnosing heart valve disease. It uses sound waves to create images of your heart and its valves. It can show your heart's size, shape, and function and your valves' structure, movement, and blood flow. It can also measure the pressure and volume of blood in your heart's chambers and vessels. There are different types of echocardiograms, such as transthoracic, transesophageal, or stress echocardiograms, depending on how the sound waves are sent and received.

- **Electrocardiogram (ECG or EKG).** This is a simple and painless test that records the electrical activity of your heart. It can show how fast and regular your heart beats and if there are any abnormal patterns or signs of damage. It can also detect arrhythmias, such as atrial fibrillation, which are common in people with heart valve disease.

- **Chest X-ray.** This is a test that uses radiation to create images of your chest, including your heart and lungs. It can show if your heart is enlarged or fluid in your lungs, which are signs of heart failure. It can also show if there are any other problems in your chest, such as pneumonia or lung cancer.

- **Cardiac MRI.** This is a test that uses a strong magnetic field and radio waves to create detailed images of your heart and its valves. It can provide more information than an echocardiogram, such as the thickness and fibrosis of your heart muscle, the extent of valve damage, and the presence of blood clots or infections. It can also measure the blood flow and pressure in your heart and vessels.

- **Exercise tests or stress tests.** These are tests that measure how your heart works under physical stress, such as walking on a treadmill or riding a stationary bike. They can show if your heart valve disease causes symptoms or affects your heart function during exercise. They can also help determine your level of fitness and your risk of having a heart attack or stroke. If you cannot exercise, you may be given a medicine that mimics the effect of exercise on your heart.

- **Cardiac catheterization.** This is an invasive test that involves inserting a thin, flexible tube called a catheter into a blood vessel, usually in your groin or wrist, and guiding it to your heart. A dye is injected through the catheter to make your heart and vessels visible on X-ray images. This test can measure the pressure and blood flow in your heart chambers and vessels and show the degree of valve narrowing or leakage. It can also detect coronary artery disease, which is a common cause or complication of heart valve disease.

These tests can help your doctor determine the best treatment plan for your heart valve disease and monitor your condition over time.

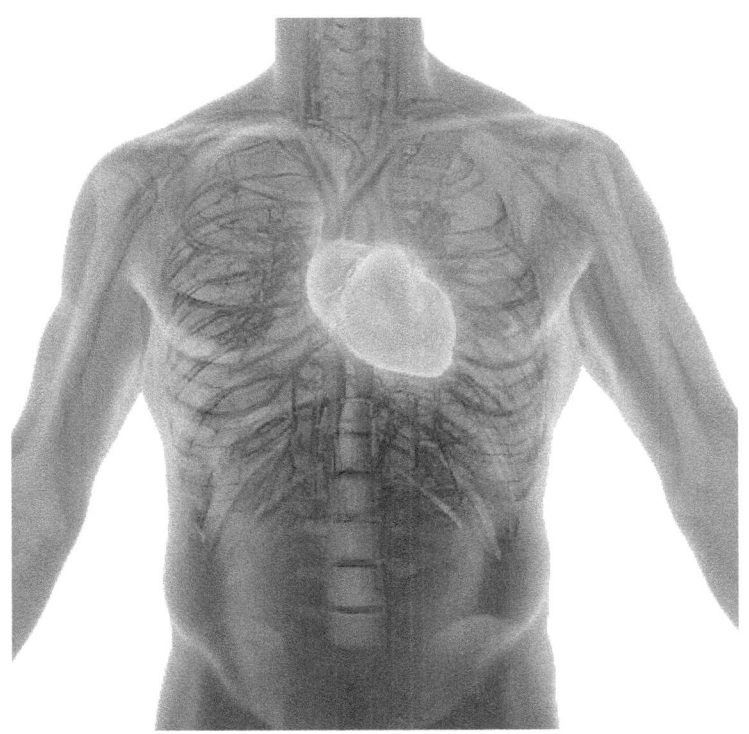

Chapter 2

Treatment Options for Faulty Heart Valves

Medications for Managing Symptoms

Heart valve disease can cause various symptoms that affect the quality of life and health of people with it. Depending on the type and severity of the valve problem, different medications may be prescribed to help relieve symptoms and prevent further complications. Some of the common medications for managing the symptoms of heart valve disease are:

- **Vasodilators.** These are medications that widen the blood vessels and lower the blood pressure. They can help reduce the heart's workload and improve the blood flow through the valves. Some examples of vasodilators are angiotensin-converting enzyme (ACE) inhibitors, angiotensin receptor blockers (ARBs), and nitrates.

- **Diuretics.** These medications increase urine output and reduce fluid retention in the body. They can help relieve the swelling, congestion, and shortness of breath caused by heart failure. Some examples of diuretics are furosemide, hydrochlorothiazide, and spironolactone.
- **Beta-blockers.** These medications slow down the heart rate and lower the blood pressure. They can help reduce the palpitations, chest pain, and anxiety caused by arrhythmias. Some examples of beta-blockers are metoprolol, atenolol, and bisoprolol.
- **Antiarrhythmics.** These medications regulate the electrical signals in the heart and restore a normal heart rhythm. They can help treat or prevent atrial fibrillation, a common arrhythmia associated with valve disease.

Some examples of antiarrhythmics are amiodarone, sotalol, and digoxin.

- **Anticoagulants.** These are medications that prevent the formation of blood clots in the heart or the blood vessels. They can help reduce the risk of stroke, heart attack, or embolism caused by valve disease. Some examples of anticoagulants are warfarin, dabigatran, and rivaroxaban.

- **Antibiotics.** These medications treat or prevent bacterial infections that can damage the valves or cause endocarditis. They can help prevent rheumatic fever, a common cause of valve disease, or treat infective endocarditis, a serious complication of valve disease. Some examples of antibiotics are penicillin, amoxicillin, and ceftriaxone.

These medications can help improve the symptoms and quality of life of people with heart valve disease.

Open-Heart Surgery for Valve Repair and Replacement

Open-heart surgery is a type of surgery that involves making a large incision in the chest and stopping the heart temporarily to access and operate on the heart valves. Open-heart surgery is the most common and traditional method of treating heart valve disease that requires surgery.

There are two main types of open-heart surgery for valve repair and replacement: valve repair and valve replacement. Valve repair is a procedure that preserves and restores the original valve's function. Valve replacement is a procedure that removes the damaged or diseased valve and replaces it with an artificial valve.

The choice between valve repair and valve replacement depends on several factors, such as the type and severity of the valve disease, the condition and durability of the valve tissue, the size and shape of the valve, the risk of infection or blood clots, the availability and compatibility of the artificial valve, and the patient's age, health, and preferences.

Valve repair is usually preferred over valve replacement as it has several advantages, such as:

- Preserving the natural structure and function of the valve and the heart
- Reducing the risk of infection, bleeding, or rejection
- Improving the long-term survival and quality of life of the patient
- Avoiding the need for lifelong blood-thinning medication

However, valve repair is only sometimes possible or effective, especially for severely damaged or calcified valves. In some cases, valve replacement may be the only or better option, as it can provide a more durable and reliable solution.

Two main types of artificial valves can be used for valve replacement: mechanical valves and biological valves. Mechanical valves are made of synthetic materials, such as metal or carbon. Biological valves are made of animal or human tissue, such as from a pig, cow, or human donor.

The choice between mechanical and biological valves also depends on several factors, such as the type and location of the valve, the durability and performance of the valve, the risk of infection or blood clots, the availability and compatibility of the valve, and the patient's age, health, and preferences.

Mechanical valves have the advantage of being durable and lasting long, usually for the rest of the patient's life. However, they have the disadvantage of being prone to forming blood clots, which can cause a stroke or embolism. Therefore, patients who receive mechanical valves need to take blood-thinning medication for the rest of their lives, which can increase the risk of bleeding and require regular monitoring and testing.

Biological valves are more natural, compatible with the body, and do not require blood-thinning medication. However, they have the disadvantage of being less durable and lasting for a shorter time, usually 10 to 15 years. Therefore, patients who receive biological valves may need to have another surgery in the future to replace the worn-out valve.

Open-heart surgery for valve repair and replacement is a major and complex operation that requires general anesthesia, a heart-lung machine, and several hours of surgery. It also involves a long and intensive recovery period, which may take several weeks or months.

The patient may need to stay in the hospital for a few days or weeks and then follow a strict medication regimen, diet, exercise, and follow-up visits. The patient may also experience side effects or complications, such as infection, bleeding, arrhythmia, or a problem with the artificial valve.

Open-heart surgery for valve repair and replacement can improve the symptoms and quality of life of people with heart valve disease, but it is not a cure.

Minimally Invasive Transcatheter Procedures

Minimally invasive transcatheter procedures are alternative methods of treating heart valve disease that use catheters (thin, flexible tubes) to access and operate on the heart valves without opening the chest or stopping the heart. Interventional cardiologists and cardiac surgeons perform these procedures in a catheterization lab.

Minimally invasive transcatheter procedures are suitable for patients who have severe valve disease that requires surgery but are considered too high-risk or ineligible for open-heart surgery due to age, health, or other factors. These procedures can also be used for patients who prefer a less invasive option or have previously had valve surgery.

There are different types of minimally invasive transcatheter procedures for valve repair and replacement, depending on the type and location of the valve. Some of the common transcatheter procedures are:

- **Transcatheter aortic valve replacement (TAVR) or transcatheter aortic valve implantation (TAVI).** This procedure replaces a narrowed or leaky aortic valve with an artificial valve made from animal tissue. The artificial valve is compressed and delivered through a catheter that is inserted through a small incision in the groin or the chest. The artificial valve is then expanded and positioned inside the diseased valve, pushing the old valve leaflets out of the way. The new valve takes over the function of regulating the blood flow from the left ventricle to the aorta.

- **Transcatheter mitral valve repair (TMVR) or transcatheter mitral valve edge-to-edge repair (TMVr).** This procedure repairs a leaky mitral valve by attaching a mechanical clip to the valve leaflets. The clip is delivered through a catheter inserted through a vein in the groin and guided to the heart. The clip clamps the valve leaflets together, reducing the leakage and improving the blood flow from the left atrium to the left ventricle. The clip stays in place permanently, allowing the valve to open and close normally.

- **Transcatheter mitral valve replacement (TMVR) or transcatheter mitral valve-in-valve (TMViV).** This procedure replaces a damaged or diseased mitral valve with an artificial valve made from animal tissue. The artificial valve is delivered through a catheter inserted through a small incision in the chest and guided to the heart. The artificial valve is then expanded and positioned inside the old valve, replacing its function of regulating the blood flow from the left atrium to the left ventricle. This procedure is mainly used for patients who have previously had mitral valve surgery and need a new valve.

- **Transcatheter pulmonary valve replacement (TPVR) or transcatheter pulmonary valve-in-valve (TPViV).** This procedure replaces a narrowed or leaky pulmonary valve with an artificial valve made from animal tissue. The artificial valve is delivered through a catheter inserted through a vein in the groin or the neck and guided to the heart. The artificial valve is then expanded and positioned inside the old valve, replacing its function of regulating the blood flow from the right ventricle to the pulmonary artery. This procedure is mainly used for patients with congenital heart defects that affect the pulmonary valve and need a new valve.

Minimally invasive transcatheter procedures have several advantages over open-heart surgery, such as:

- Shorter and less painful recovery time
- Less risk of infection, bleeding, or complications
- No need for general anesthesia or a heart-lung machine
- No need for a large chest incision or sternotomy
- No need for lifelong blood-thinning medication (except for some mechanical valves)

However, minimally invasive transcatheter procedures also have some limitations and challenges, such as:

- Higher cost and limited availability.
- Less durability and performance of some artificial valves.

- Higher risk of stroke, vascular injury, or valve leakage.
- Need for regular monitoring and testing of the artificial valve.
- Need for repeat procedures in some cases.

Minimally invasive transcatheter procedures can improve the symptoms and quality of life of people with heart valve disease, but they are not a cure. The patient will still need to take care of their heart and monitor their condition regularly. The patient may also need to make lifestyle changes, such as quitting smoking, eating a healthy diet, managing stress, and avoiding strenuous activities.

Choosing the Right Treatment Approach

Choosing the right treatment approach for your heart valve disease can be a difficult and complex decision. There are many factors to consider, such as the type and severity of your valve problem, the risks and benefits of each option, your personal preferences and values, and your overall health and life expectancy.

The main goal of treatment is to improve your symptoms and quality of life, prevent further complications, and prolong your survival. However, each treatment option has advantages and disadvantages and may not be suitable or effective for everyone. Therefore, it is important to discuss your options with your doctor and understand the pros and cons of each option.

Some of the questions you may want to ask your doctor are:

- How severe is my valve disease, and how is it affecting my heart function and health?
- What are the possible outcomes and complications of my valve disease if left untreated or treated with medication only?
- What are the different types of surgery or transcatheter procedures available for my valve problem, and how do they work?
- What are the risks and benefits of each option, and how do they compare to each other?

- How likely can each option improve my symptoms and quality of life, prevent further complications, and prolong my survival?
- How durable and reliable is each option, and what are the chances of needing another procedure in the future?
- How long and intensive is the recovery period for each option, and what are the possible side effects or complications during or after the procedure?
- How will each option affect my lifestyle, activities, and medication needs?
- What are the costs and availability of each option, and will my insurance cover them?
- What are the preferences and experiences of other patients with similar valve problems and treatments?
- What are my values and goals regarding my health and quality of life?

You may also want to seek a second opinion from another doctor or a heart valve specialist, especially if you have doubts or concerns about your diagnosis or treatment plan. You may also want to involve your family and friends in decision-making, as they can provide support and advice.

Ultimately, the decision is yours based on the best available information and your personal preferences. Choose the option that you feel most comfortable and confident with and that aligns with your values and goals. You should also be prepared to accept the possible outcomes and consequences of your choice and be ready to follow the instructions and recommendations of your doctor and health care team.

Choosing the right treatment approach for your heart valve disease can be a challenging and stressful process; however, it can also be a rewarding and empowering one. By being well-informed and actively involved in your decision-making process, you can make the best choice for your health and well-being.

Chapter 3

Preparing for Heart Valve Surgery

Finding the Right Cardiac Surgeon

Finding the right cardiac surgeon is important in preparing for heart valve surgery. A cardiac surgeon is a doctor who specializes in performing surgery on the heart and its valves. A good cardiac surgeon can improve your chances of successful surgery and a smooth recovery.

There are several factors to consider when choosing a cardiac surgeon, such as:

- **Credentials and experience.** You should look for a cardiac surgeon who is board-certified in cardiothoracic surgery and has extensive training and experience in performing the type of surgery you need. You should also check the surgeon's reputation, ratings, and reviews from other patients and sources. You can find this information on Healthgrades.com, The Society of Thoracic Surgeons, or your state's Department of Health.

- **Hospital quality and location.** Choose a cardiac surgeon who works at a hospital with high-quality cardiac surgery standards and outcomes. You can compare the performance and ratings of different hospitals on websites such as Healthgrades.com or Medicare.gov. You should also consider the location of the hospital and how convenient and accessible it is for you and your family.

- **Communication style and personality.** Choose a cardiac surgeon who listens to you, answers your questions, explains your options, and respects your preferences and values. You should feel comfortable and confident with your surgeon and trust their judgment and expertise. You can assess the surgeon's communication style and personality during consultation or by reading patient reviews.

- **Insurance coverage and cost.** Choose a cardiac surgeon who accepts your insurance plan and charges reasonable fees for the surgery and follow-up care. You should also ask about the estimated cost of the surgery and what it includes, such as hospital fees, anesthesia fees, and postoperative care. Also, inquire about any available financial assistance or payment plans.

To find the right cardiac surgeon, you can start by getting referrals from your primary care doctor or cardiologist, who can recommend surgeons they trust and work with. You can also ask your family, friends, or other healthcare professionals for their suggestions. You can then research the surgeons' credentials, experience, and reviews online and narrow your list. You can then contact the surgeons' offices and schedule a consultation to meet and interview them. You can also seek a second opinion from another surgeon if you have any doubts or concerns.

What to Expect Before, During, and After Surgery

Heart valve surgery is a major operation that requires careful preparation and recovery. Knowing what to expect before, during, and after surgery can help you feel more prepared and confident. Here are some general guidelines, but you should always follow your doctor's specific instructions and recommendations.

Before surgery.

Before surgery, you must undergo tests and evaluations to ensure you are ready. These may include blood tests, chest X-rays, electrocardiograms, echocardiograms, cardiac catheterization, and other imaging tests. You will also meet with your surgeon, anesthesiologist, and other surgical team members to discuss the details and risks of the surgery and to sign a consent form.

You will need to stop taking certain medications, such as blood thinners, anti-inflammatory drugs, or herbal supplements, a few days or weeks before surgery, as they may increase the risk of bleeding or interfere with the surgery. You will also need to fast (not eat or drink anything) for at least eight hours before surgery to prevent nausea or vomiting. You may be given some medications to take before surgery, such as antibiotics, to prevent infection.

You should pack a bag with some personal items you will need during your hospital stay, such as comfortable clothes, slippers, toiletries, glasses, hearing aids, dentures, and a list of your medications and allergies. You should also arrange for someone to drive you to and from the hospital to help you with your daily activities after surgery. You should not smoke, drink alcohol, or use any recreational drugs before surgery, as they may affect your recovery.

During surgery.

On the day of surgery, you will be admitted to the hospital and taken to a preoperative area, where you will change into a hospital gown and have an intravenous (IV) line inserted into your arm. You will also have some monitors attached to your chest, arms, and legs to measure your heart rate, blood pressure, oxygen level, and other vital signs. You will then be taken to the operating room, where you will receive general anesthesia, which will make you fall asleep and feel no pain during the surgery.

The surgery will last for several hours, depending on the type and complexity of the procedure. The surgeon will make an incision in your chest, usually along the breastbone (sternum), to access your heart. You will be connected to a heart-lung machine, which will take over the function of your heart and lungs during the surgery. The surgeon will then repair or replace your damaged or diseased valve using either your tissue, an artificial valve, or a biological valve from an animal or human donor. The surgeon will then close the incision with stitches or staples and cover it with a bandage. You will be disconnected from the heart-lung machine, and your heart will resume its normal function.

After surgery.

After surgery, you will be taken to a recovery room or an intensive care unit (ICU), where you will be closely monitored for any complications, such as bleeding, infection, arrhythmia, or a problem with the new valve. You will have some tubes and wires attached to your body, such as a breathing tube, a chest tube, a urinary catheter, and an arterial line. You will also receive some medications, such as painkillers, antibiotics, and blood thinners, through your IV line. You will gradually wake up from the anesthesia, and the breathing tube will be removed when you can breathe on your own.

Depending on your condition and recovery, you will stay in the hospital for several days or weeks. You will be moved to a regular room, where you will continue to receive care and support from your medical team. You will be encouraged to get up, walk, and do breathing exercises to prevent blood clots, pneumonia, and muscle weakness.

You will also have tests and evaluations, such as chest X-rays, electrocardiograms, echocardiograms, and blood tests, to check your heart function and healing. You will be given some instructions and education on how to care for your incision, manage your pain, take your medications, and follow a healthy diet and lifestyle. You will also be referred to a cardiac rehabilitation program, which will help you regain your strength and endurance and reduce your risk of future heart problems.

Recovery Process and Rehabilitation

The recovery process and rehabilitation are essential to your treatment after heart valve surgery. They can help you heal faster, prevent complications, and improve your heart function and quality of life. The recovery process and rehabilitation may vary depending on the type and extent of your surgery, overall health, and individual needs and goals. Here are some general guidelines, but you should always follow your doctor's specific instructions and recommendations.

Recovery process.

The recovery process begins right after your surgery until you are fully healed and ready to resume your normal activities. The recovery process may involve the following stages:

- **Hospital stay.** You will stay in the hospital for a few days or weeks after your surgery, depending on your condition and progress. You will be closely monitored and cared for by your medical team, who will check your vital signs, wound healing, heart function, and blood tests. You will also receive medications, such as painkillers, antibiotics, and blood thinners, to help you recover and prevent infection or blood clots. You will be encouraged to get up, walk, and do breathing exercises to prevent pneumonia, muscle weakness, and blood clots. You will also receive education and counseling on how to care for yourself at home, take your medications, and follow a healthy lifestyle.

- **Home care.** You will be discharged from the hospital when you are stable and ready to continue your recovery at home. You will need someone to drive you home and help you with your daily activities for a few weeks. You must also follow some precautions and restrictions, such as avoiding lifting heavy objects, driving, or bathing until your doctor allows you. You must care for your incision, keep it clean and dry, and watch for any signs of infection, such as redness, swelling, or pus. You will also need to take your medications as prescribed and monitor your symptoms, such as chest pain, shortness of breath, or fever. You will need to visit your doctor regularly for follow-up appointments, where your doctor will check your wound, heart function, and blood tests.

- **Recovery period.** The recovery period is when you can heal completely and return to your normal activities. The recovery period may vary from person to person; however, it usually takes about 4 to 8 weeks for open-heart surgery and 2 to 4 weeks for minimally invasive surgery. During this time, you will gradually increase your activity level, as guided by your doctor and cardiac rehabilitation team. You will also need to make lifestyle changes, such as quitting smoking, eating a heart-healthy diet, managing stress, and avoiding alcohol or caffeine. You will also need to be aware of the signs and symptoms of complications, such as stroke, heart attack, or valve problems, and seek immediate medical attention if they occur.

Rehabilitation.

Rehabilitation is a program that helps you improve your physical, mental, and emotional well-being after heart valve surgery. Rehabilitation may start during your hospital stay and continue after you go home until you reach optimal functioning and quality of life. Rehabilitation may involve the following components:

- **Cardiac rehabilitation.** Cardiac rehabilitation is a supervised program that helps you improve your heart health and fitness after heart valve surgery. Cardiac rehabilitation may include exercise training, education, counseling, and support. Cardiac rehabilitation can help you regain strength and endurance, reduce the risk of future heart problems, and enhance your confidence and well-being. Cardiac rehabilitation is usually offered at a hospital or a clinic, where you will work with a team of health professionals, such as cardiologists, nurses, physiotherapists, and dietitians. Cardiac rehabilitation may last for several weeks or months, depending on your needs and goals.

- **Physical therapy.** Physical therapy is a treatment that helps you restore your mobility and function after heart valve surgery. Physical therapy may include exercises, stretches, massage, heat, cold, or electrical stimulation. Physical therapy can help you improve your range of motion, flexibility, balance, and coordination. Physical therapy may be provided by a physiotherapist or a physical therapist, either at a hospital, a clinic, or at home. Depending on your condition and progress, physical therapy may last a few weeks or months.

- **Occupational therapy.** Occupational therapy is a treatment that helps you perform your daily activities and tasks after heart valve surgery. Occupational therapy may include training, equipment, or modifications. Occupational therapy can help you improve your skills, such as dressing, bathing, cooking, or working. Occupational therapy may be provided by an occupational therapist at a hospital, clinic, or home. Depending on your needs and goals, occupational therapy may last a few weeks or months.

- **Psychological therapy.** Psychological therapy is a treatment that helps you cope with your emotional and mental health issues after heart valve surgery. Psychological therapy may include counseling, psychotherapy, or medication. Psychological therapy can help you deal with your feelings, such as anxiety, depression, anger, or grief. Psychological therapy may also help you adjust to your new situation, such as living with an artificial valve, taking medications, or making lifestyle changes. A psychologist, a psychiatrist, or a counselor at a hospital, clinic, or home may provide psychological therapy. Depending on your needs and goals, psychological therapy may last for a few weeks or months.

The recovery process and rehabilitation are important steps in your treatment after heart valve surgery. They can help you heal faster, prevent complications, and improve your heart function and quality of life. The recovery process and rehabilitation may vary depending on the type and extent of your surgery, overall health, and individual needs and goals.

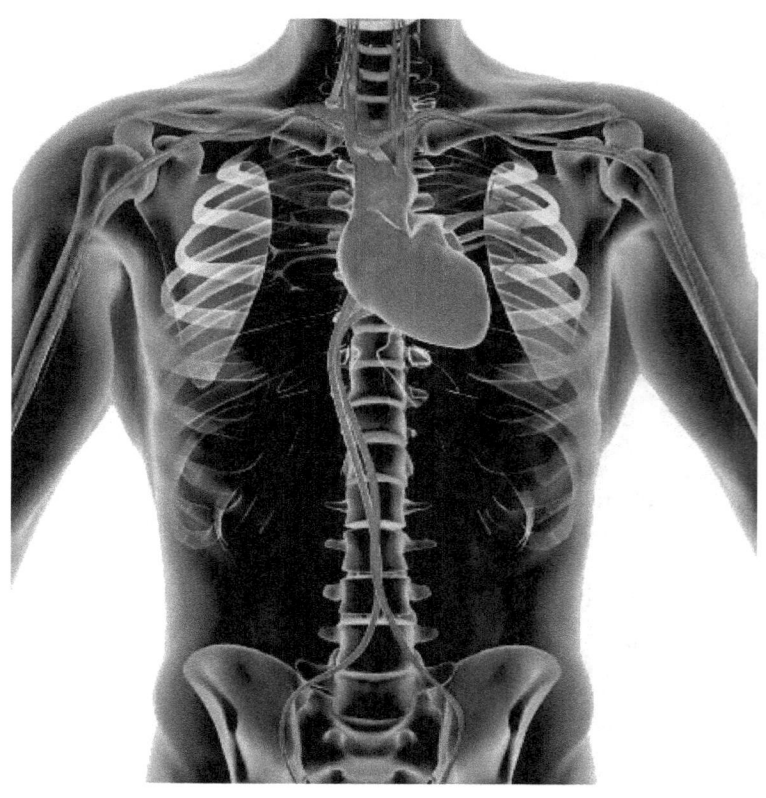

Chapter 4

Life After Heart Valve Surgery

Follow-Up Care and Monitoring

Follow-up care and monitoring are essential to your treatment after heart valve surgery. They can help you prevent complications, detect problems, and optimize your heart function and quality of life.

Follow-up care and monitoring may vary depending on the type and extent of your surgery, overall health, and individual needs and goals. Here are some general guidelines, but you should always follow your doctor's specific instructions and recommendations.

Follow-up care.

Follow-up care is the care you receive after surgery to help you recover and adjust to your new situation. Follow-up care may involve the following aspects:

- **Medications.** You will need to take some medications after your surgery, such as blood thinners, antibiotics, antiarrhythmics, and heart failure drugs. These medications can help you prevent infection, blood clots, arrhythmia, and heart failure. You must take your medications as prescribed and monitor your symptoms and side effects. You will also need regular blood tests, such as INR, to check the effectiveness and safety of your medications. You should not stop or change your medications without consulting your doctor.
- **Wound care.** You must care for your surgical incision and keep it clean and dry. You must change your dressing as instructed and watch for any signs of infection, such as redness, swelling, pain, or pus. You should avoid touching, scratching, or picking at your

wound. You should also avoid applying creams, lotions, or ointments to your wound unless your doctor advises. You should report any problems or concerns to your doctor immediately.

- **Activity and exercise.** You will need to gradually resume your physical activity and exercise after your surgery, as guided by your doctor and cardiac rehabilitation team. You must start with light activities, such as walking, and increase your intensity and duration. You must avoid strenuous activities, such as lifting, pushing, or pulling heavy objects until your doctor allows you. You must also avoid activities that may pressure your chest, such as coughing, sneezing, or straining. You should listen to your body and stop or rest if you feel tired, dizzy, or short of breath. You should also drink plenty of fluids and wear comfortable and loose-fitting clothes and shoes.

- **Diet and nutrition.** You must follow a heart-healthy diet after your surgery to help you control your weight, blood pressure, cholesterol, and blood sugar. A heart-healthy diet is low in saturated fat, trans fat, salt, and added sugar and high in fruits, vegetables, whole grains, lean protein, and healthy fats. You will also need to limit your intake of alcohol, caffeine, and tobacco, as they may affect your heart function and medication effectiveness. You should consult your doctor or a dietitian for more specific advice and guidance.

- **Lifestyle and habits.** You must make some lifestyle changes and adopt healthy habits after your surgery to help improve your heart health and well-being. These may include quitting smoking, managing stress, getting enough sleep, and caring for mental and emotional health. You should also seek support from your family, friends, or other sources, such as support groups, counselors, or online communities. You should also follow your doctor's advice on driving, traveling, working, and sexual activity.

Monitoring.

Monitoring checks your heart function and valve performance after surgery to detect any problems or complications. Monitoring may involve the following methods:

- **Physical examination.** You will need regular physical examinations by your doctor, who will check your vital signs, such as blood pressure, heart rate, and temperature, and listen to your heart sounds and lungs. Your doctor will also ask about your symptoms, medications, and lifestyle.

- **Echocardiography.** You will need to have regular echocardiograms, which are ultrasound tests that show the structure and function of your heart and valves. Echocardiograms can help you measure the size and shape of your heart chambers, the thickness and movement of your heart walls, the blood flow and pressure in your heart and vessels, and the opening and closing of your valves. Echocardiograms can also help you detect any problems or complications, such as valve leakage, narrowing, infection, or thrombosis.

- **Electrocardiography.** You will need regular electrocardiograms to measure your heart's electrical activity. Electrocardiograms can help you monitor your heart rhythm and rate and detect any arrhythmias, such as atrial fibrillation, ventricular tachycardia, or heart block. Electrocardiograms can also help you assess the effect of your medications on your heart.

- **Chest X-ray.** You may need to have occasional chest X-rays, which are tests that show images of your chest, lungs, and heart. Chest X-rays can help you check for any fluid accumulation, infection, or inflammation in your lungs, as well as any changes in the size or shape of your heart.

- **Blood tests.** You may need periodic blood tests, which measure the levels of different substances in your blood. Blood tests can help you monitor your kidney and liver function, blood count, electrolytes, inflammation markers, and infection indicators. Blood tests can also help you adjust your medication dosage, such as blood thinners or heart failure drugs.

Follow-up care and monitoring are essential to your treatment after heart valve surgery. They can help you prevent complications, detect problems, and optimize your heart function and quality of life.

Managing Pain and Discomfort

Managing pain and discomfort is an integral part of your recovery after heart valve surgery. Pain and discomfort can affect your physical, mental, and emotional well-being and interfere with healing and rehabilitation. Therefore, you should not ignore or endure your pain and discomfort but seek help and relief from your doctor and health care team.

The following information will help you understand the causes and types of pain and discomfort you may experience after heart valve surgery, describe how you can help your doctors and nurses assess and treat your pain and discomfort, and empower you to take an active role in making choices about pain and discomfort management.

Causes and types of pain and discomfort.

After heart valve surgery, you may experience different pain and discomfort depending on the sensation's location, intensity, duration, and frequency. Some of the common causes and types of pain and discomfort are:

- **Incision pain:** You may feel pain, pressure, or burning at the site of your surgical incision, especially when you move, cough, or breathe deeply. This is expected as your wound is healing and your nerves regenerate. Incision pain usually improves as the wound heals and the inflammation subsides.

- **Muscle pain:** You may feel pain, stiffness, or soreness in your chest, back, neck, or shoulders. This is due to the trauma and manipulation of your muscles and bones during surgery and the prolonged immobility and inactivity after surgery. Muscle pain usually improves with gentle movement, stretching, and massage.

- **Nerve pain:** You may feel pain, numbness, tingling, or shooting sensations in your chest, arms, or legs. This is due to the damage or irritation of your nerves during surgery or the compression of your nerves by swelling or inflammation. Nerve pain usually improves as the nerves heal, and the swelling decreases.

- **Chest tube pain:** You may feel pain or discomfort from the chest tubes inserted in your chest to drain fluid, blood, and air during and after surgery. Chest tube pain usually improves as the tubes are removed and the holes heal.
- **Throat pain:** You may feel a sore throat from the breathing tube inserted in your mouth or nose during surgery. Throat pain usually improves with lozenges, ice chips, or gargling.
- **Headache:** You may feel pain or pressure in your head from the anesthesia, medications, dehydration, or lack of sleep. Headaches usually improve with rest, hydration, and painkillers.

Assessment and treatment of pain and discomfort.

Doctors and nurses will assess and treat your pain and discomfort using various methods and tools after heart valve surgery. Some of the common methods and tools are:

- **Pain scale:** You will be asked to rate your pain on a scale of 0 to 10, with 0 being no pain and 10 being the worst pain imaginable. This will help your doctors and nurses measure the intensity of your pain and the effectiveness of your treatment. You should be honest and consistent when rating your pain and reporting any changes or concerns.

- **Pain medication:** You will be given pain medication to help you relieve your pain and discomfort. Pain medication has different types and routes, such as pills, injections, patches, or pumps. Your doctors and nurses will choose your best type and route based on your condition, preference, and response. You should take your pain medication as prescribed and monitor your symptoms and side effects. You should not stop or change your pain medication without consulting your doctor.

- **Non-pharmacological methods:** You may also use non-pharmacological methods to help you cope with pain and discomfort, such as ice, heat, massage, relaxation, distraction, or music. These methods can complement your pain medication and enhance your comfort and well-being. You should consult your doctor or nurse before using non-pharmacological methods and follow their instructions and recommendations.

Choices and preferences for pain and discomfort management.

You have the right and responsibility to participate in your pain and discomfort management after heart valve surgery. You can choose and express your preferences based on the best available information and your values and goals. Some of the choices and preferences you can make are:

- **Setting a pain goal:** You can set a realistic and acceptable pain goal for yourself, such as a pain score of 3 or less or being able to perform certain activities without pain. This will help you and your doctors and nurses evaluate your progress and adjust your treatment. You should communicate your pain goal to your doctors and nurses and update it as needed.

- **Choosing a pain medication:** You can select one that suits your needs and preferences, such as the type, route, dose, and frequency. You should discuss the pros and cons of each option with your doctor or nurse and consider the effectiveness, safety, convenience, and cost of each option. You should also inform your doctor or nurse of any allergies, intolerances, or interactions with any medication.

- **Using non-pharmacological methods:** You can use non-pharmacological methods that work for you and make you feel comfortable, such as ice, heat, massage, relaxation, distraction, or music. You should explore different methods and find out what helps you the most. You should also ask your doctor or nurse for guidance and support on using these methods safely and effectively.

- **Seeking help and support:** You can seek help and support from your doctors, nurses, and other healthcare professionals, as well as your family, friends, or other sources, such as support groups, counselors, or online communities. You should not hesitate or be afraid to ask for help or support; they can make a difference in your recovery and well-being. You should also give feedback and appreciation to those who help and support you.

Managing pain and discomfort is an integral part of your recovery after heart valve surgery. Pain and discomfort can affect your physical, mental, and emotional well-being and interfere with healing and rehabilitation. Therefore, you should not ignore or endure your pain and discomfort but seek help and relief from your doctor and health care team. You should also take an active role in your pain and discomfort management, make choices, and express preferences that suit your needs and goals.

Returning to Normal Activities

Returning to normal activities is one of the main goals of your recovery after heart valve surgery. Normal activities are the things you do in your daily life, such as work, leisure, hobbies, and social interactions. Returning to normal activities can help you improve your physical, mental, and emotional well-being and enhance your quality of life.

However, returning to normal activities may pose challenges and risks, such as fatigue, stress, or complications. Therefore, you should not rush or force yourself to return to normal activities but follow a gradual and safe process guided by your doctor and health care team.

The following information will help you understand the benefits and barriers of returning to normal activities after heart valve surgery, describe how you can plan and prepare for returning to normal activities, and empower you to make choices and express preferences that suit your needs and goals.

Benefits and barriers to returning to normal activities.

Returning to normal activities after heart valve surgery can have many benefits, such as:

- Improving your physical health and fitness by strengthening your heart, muscles, and bones and preventing weight gain, diabetes, and other chronic diseases.
- Improving your mental and emotional health by reducing your anxiety, depression, and boredom and increasing your confidence, self-esteem, and happiness.
- Improving your social and family relationships by reconnecting with your loved ones, friends, and colleagues and participating in meaningful and enjoyable activities.
- Improving your personal and professional development by resuming your education, career, or hobbies and pursuing your interests and goals.

However, returning to normal activities after heart valve surgery may also have some barriers, such as:

- Experiencing fatigue, pain, or discomfort may limit your energy and ability to perform certain activities.
- Facing stress, pressure, or expectations may overwhelm or discourage you from returning to certain activities.
- Encountering complications like infection, bleeding, arrhythmia, or a valve problem may require you to stop or modify certain activities.
- Lacking support, guidance, or resources may hinder or delay your return to certain activities.

Plan and prepare for returning to normal activities

To overcome the barriers and enjoy the benefits of returning to normal activities after heart valve surgery, you need to plan and prepare for the process with the help of your doctor and healthcare team. You can use the following steps to plan and prepare for returning to normal activities:

- **Assess your current situation.** You can evaluate your current physical, mental, and emotional condition and identify your strengths and weaknesses, needs and challenges, and priorities and preferences. You can also review your pre-surgery activities and determine which ones are important and meaningful to you and which ones are not.

- **Set realistic and achievable goals.** You can set short-term and long-term goals for returning to normal activities based on your current situation, values, and aspirations. You can make your goals specific, measurable, attainable, relevant, and time-bound and write them down or share them with someone. You can also monitor your progress and celebrate your achievements.

- **Follow a gradual and safe process.** You can follow a gradual and safe process for returning to normal activities, as guided by your doctor and health care team. You can start with low-intensity and low-frequency activities, such as walking, reading, or watching TV, and gradually increase your intensity and frequency as your condition and tolerance improve. You can also follow general precautions and restrictions, such as avoiding lifting heavy objects, driving, or bathing until your doctor allows you. You can also listen to your body and stop or rest if you feel tired, dizzy, or short of breath.

- **Seek help and support.** You can seek help and support from your doctor and healthcare team, as well as from your family, friends, or other sources, such as support groups, counselors, or online communities. You can ask for help or advice on returning to normal activities and coping with any difficulties or challenges. You can also give feedback and appreciation to those who help and support you.

Choices and preferences for returning to normal activities

You have the right and responsibility to participate in your return to normal activities after heart valve surgery. You can choose and express preferences based on the best available information and your values and goals. Some of the choices and preferences you can make are as follows:

- **Choosing the activities you want to return to.** You can choose the activities you want to return to based on your interests, passions, and goals. You can also choose beneficial and enjoyable activities and avoid harmful or stressful ones. You can also try new activities or modify existing ones to suit your needs and abilities.

- **Choosing the pace and timing of your return to normal activities.** You can choose the pace and timing of your return to normal activities based on your condition, progress, and comfort. You can also choose a pace and timing that are realistic and flexible and adjust them as needed. You can also respect your limits and not compare yourself to others or your pre-surgery self.

- **Choosing the people you want to return to normal activities with.** You can choose the people you want to return to normal activities with based on your relationships, expectations, and compatibility. You can also choose supportive and encouraging people and avoid those who are negative or demanding. You can also communicate your needs and preferences to the people you return to normal activities with and respect their needs and preferences as well.

Returning to normal activities is one of the main goals of your recovery after heart valve surgery. Normal activities are the things you do in your daily life, such as work, leisure, hobbies, and social interactions. Returning to normal activities can help you improve your physical, mental, and emotional well-being and enhance your quality of life.

Diet and Lifestyle Guidelines

Diet and lifestyle guidelines are important to your treatment and prevention after heart valve surgery. Diet and lifestyle guidelines can help you improve your heart function and health, reduce your risk of complications and recurrence, and enhance your quality of life. Diet and lifestyle guidelines may vary depending on the type and extent of your surgery, overall health, and individual needs and goals. Here are some general guidelines, but you should always follow your doctor's specific instructions and recommendations.

Diet guidelines.

Diet guidelines recommend what and how much you should eat and drink after heart valve surgery. Diet guidelines can help you control your weight, blood pressure, cholesterol, and blood sugar and prevent infection, blood clots, and inflammation. Diet guidelines may involve the following aspects:

- **Calories.** Calories are the units of energy that you get from food and drink. You need calories to fuel your body and support your recovery, but not too many or too few. You should eat enough calories to maintain a healthy weight, as being overweight or underweight can strain your heart and increase your risk of complications. You should consult your doctor or a dietitian for your calorie needs and monitor your weight regularly.

- **Protein.** Protein is the nutrient that helps build and repair your muscles, tissues, and organs, including your heart and valves. You need protein to heal your wound, prevent infection, and support your immune system. You should eat enough protein to meet your needs, but not too much or too little. You should choose lean and high-quality protein sources, such as fish, poultry, eggs, dairy, soy, nuts, and legumes. You should avoid processed and fatty meats, such as bacon, sausage, or ham, as they are high in saturated fat, salt, and additives.

- **Carbohydrates.** Carbohydrates are the nutrients that provide energy for your body and brain. You need carbohydrates to fuel your activity and recovery, but not too much or too little. You should choose complex and high-fiber carbohydrates, such as whole grains, fruits, vegetables, and legumes. You should avoid simple and refined carbohydrates, such as white bread, white rice, pastries, candies, and sodas, as they are low in nutrients and fiber and high in sugar and calories.

- **Fat.** Fat is the nutrient that helps absorb vitamins, hormones, and cell membranes. You need fat to support your health and recovery, but not too much or too little. You should choose healthy and unsaturated fats, such as olive oil, avocado, nuts, seeds, and fish. You should avoid unhealthy and saturated fats, such as butter, lard, cream, cheese, and fatty meats, as they are high in cholesterol and calories and can clog your arteries and damage your heart. You should also limit your intake of trans fats, which are artificial fats found in some processed and fried foods, such as margarine, cakes, cookies, and chips, as they harm your heart and health.

- **Vitamins and minerals.** Vitamins and minerals are the nutrients that help regulate your body's functions and processes, such as blood clotting, wound healing, and immune response. You need vitamins and minerals to support your health and recovery, but not too much or too little. You should get most of your vitamins and minerals from food and drink, especially fruits, vegetables, and whole grains, which are rich in antioxidants, phytochemicals, and fiber. You should avoid taking supplements unless prescribed by your doctor, as some supplements may interfere with your medications or cause side effects. You should also be careful with your intake of vitamin K, which is found in green leafy vegetables such as spinach, kale, or broccoli, as it can affect the effectiveness of your blood thinners. You should consult your doctor or a dietitian for your vitamin and mineral needs and monitor your blood tests regularly.

- **Fluids.** Fluids are the liquids that help hydrate your body and flush out toxins and waste. You need fluids to support your health and recovery, but not too much or too little. You should drink enough fluids to keep your urine clear or pale yellow and prevent dehydration, constipation, or kidney stones. You should choose water as your main source of fluids and limit your intake of other beverages, such as juice, milk, coffee, tea, or alcohol, as they may contain sugar, calories, caffeine, or ethanol, affecting your heart function and medication effectiveness. You should also limit your salt intake, which is found in table salt, soy sauce, canned foods, and processed foods, as it can cause fluid retention, high blood pressure, and heart failure. You should consult your doctor or a dietitian for your fluid and salt needs and monitor your symptoms and signs of fluid overload, such as swelling, shortness of breath, or weight gain.

Lifestyle guidelines.

Lifestyle guidelines recommend how you should live and behave after heart valve surgery. Lifestyle guidelines can help you improve your physical, mental, and emotional well-being and prevent complications and recurrences. Lifestyle guidelines may involve the following aspects:

- **Activity and exercise.** Activity and exercise are the movements that help strengthen your heart, muscles, and bones and improve your blood circulation, oxygen delivery, and metabolism. You need activity and exercise to support your recovery and health, but not too much or too little. You should follow a gradual and safe process for resuming your activity and exercise, as guided by your doctor and cardiac rehabilitation team. You should start with low-intensity and low-frequency activities, such as walking, and gradually increase your intensity and frequency as your condition and tolerance improve. You should avoid strenuous and high-impact activities, such as running, jumping, or lifting heavy objects, until your doctor allows you. You should also follow some general precautions and restrictions, such as avoiding activities that may pressure your chest, such as coughing, sneezing, or straining. You should listen to your body and stop or rest if you feel tired, dizzy, or short of breath. You should also drink plenty of fluids and wear comfortable and loose-fitting clothes and shoes.

- **Smoking and alcohol.** Smoking and alcohol are habits that harm your heart, lungs, and blood vessels and increase your risk of complications and recurrence. You should quit smoking and limit your alcohol intake after heart valve surgery, as they can affect your heart function and medication effectiveness. You should seek help and support from your doctor and healthcare team, as well as from your family, friends, or other sources, such as support groups, counselors, or online communities, to help you quit smoking and limit your alcohol intake. You should also avoid exposure to secondhand smoke, which can also harm your heart and health.

- **Stress and emotions.** Stress and emotions are the feelings and reactions that affect your mood, behavior, and well-being. You may experience stress and emotions after heart valve surgery, such as anxiety, depression, anger, or grief, as you cope with your condition, surgery, and recovery. After heart valve surgery, you should manage your stress and emotions, as they can affect your heart function and health. You should seek help and support from your doctor and healthcare team and your family, friends, or other sources, such as support groups, counselors, or online communities, to help you cope with your stress and emotions. You should also practice relaxation techniques, such as breathing, meditation, or yoga, to help you calm your mind and body. You should also engage in enjoyable activities, such as hobbies, music, or reading, to help you distract yourself and lift your mood.

- **Education and awareness.** Education and awareness are the knowledge and understanding that help you make informed decisions and take action for your health and recovery. You should educate and become aware of yourself after heart valve surgery, as it can help you improve your outcomes and quality of life. You should seek information and guidance from your doctor, health care team, and other reliable sources, such as books, websites, or organizations, to help you learn about your condition, surgery, and recovery. You should also be aware of the signs and symptoms of complications, such as infection, bleeding, arrhythmia, or a valve problem, and seek immediate medical attention if they occur. You should also be aware of the factors that can affect your heart function and health, such as diet, lifestyle, medications, and follow-up care, and follow your doctor's instructions and recommendations.

Diet and lifestyle guidelines are important to your treatment and prevention after heart valve surgery. Diet and lifestyle guidelines can help you improve your heart function and health, reduce your risk of complications and recurrence, and enhance your quality of life. Diet and lifestyle guidelines may vary depending on the type and extent of your surgery, overall health, and individual needs and goals.

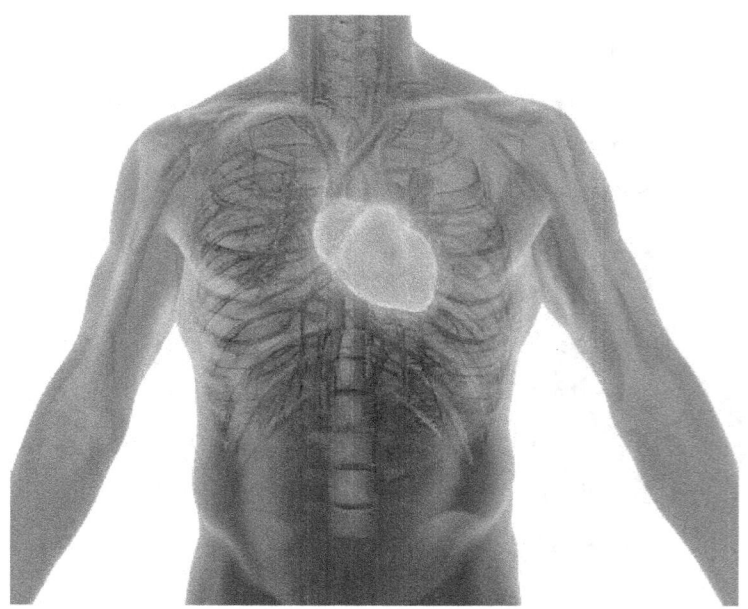

Chapter 5

Improving Your Cardiovascular Health

Managing Heart Disease Risk Factors

Managing heart disease risk factors is one of the most effective ways to improve cardiovascular health and prevent complications and recurrence after heart valve surgery. Heart disease risk factors are the conditions or behaviors that increase your chance of developing or worsening heart disease.

Some heart disease risk factors are modifiable, meaning you can change or control them, such as smoking, high blood pressure, or high cholesterol. Some heart disease risk factors are non-modifiable, meaning you cannot change or control them, such as age, gender, or family history.

The following information will help you understand the common heart disease risk factors, describe how you can measure and monitor your heart disease risk factors, and empower you to take action and make choices to reduce your heart disease risk factors.

Common heart disease risk factors

According to the American Heart Association, the common heart disease risk factors are:

- **High blood pressure.** High blood pressure, also called hypertension, is a condition that occurs when the force of blood against the walls of your arteries is too high. High blood pressure can damage your arteries, heart, and other organs and increase your risk of heart attack, stroke, heart failure, and kidney disease. High blood pressure often has no signs or symptoms, so checking your blood pressure regularly is essential.
- **High blood cholesterol.** High blood cholesterol, also called hypercholesterolemia,

is a condition that occurs when you have too much cholesterol in your blood. Cholesterol is a waxy, fat-like substance needed to make hormones, vitamin D, and bile acids. However, too much cholesterol can build up in your arteries and form plaques, which can narrow or block the blood flow to your heart and other organs and increase your risk of heart attack, stroke, and peripheral artery disease. High blood cholesterol usually has no signs or symptoms, so checking your blood cholesterol levels regularly is important.

- **Smoking.** Smoking, or using any tobacco products, is a habit that harms your heart, lungs, and blood vessels and increases your risk of heart disease and many other diseases. Smoking damages the lining of your arteries reduces the amount of oxygen in your blood, increases your blood pressure and heart rate, makes your blood more likely to clot, and lowers your HDL (good) cholesterol. Smoking also exposes you and others to harmful chemicals, such as nicotine, carbon monoxide, and tar. Smoking can also affect the effectiveness of your medications and the healing of your wound after heart valve surgery.

- **Diabetes.** Diabetes, also called diabetes mellitus, is a condition that occurs when your blood sugar (glucose) level is too high. Glucose is the main energy source for your cells and comes from the food you eat. Insulin is a hormone that helps glucose get into your cells. If you have diabetes, your body either does not make enough insulin, cannot use the insulin it makes, or both. As a result, glucose stays in your blood and can cause serious health problems. Diabetes can damage your heart, blood vessels, nerves, eyes, and kidneys and increase your risk of heart disease, stroke, and kidney disease. Diabetes can also affect the healing of your wound after heart valve surgery.
- **Obesity.** Obesity, also called overweight, is a condition that occurs when you have too much body fat. Obesity can affect your health in many ways and increase your risk of heart disease and many other diseases. Obesity can

raise your blood pressure, cholesterol, and blood sugar levels and cause inflammation and oxidative stress. Obesity can also make it harder for you to breathe, move, and exercise and affect your self-esteem and mental health. Obesity can also affect the success of your heart valve surgery's success and recovery.

- **Physical inactivity.** Physical inactivity, also called a sedentary lifestyle, is a habit that involves little or no physical activity or exercise. Physical inactivity can affect your health in many ways and increase your risk of heart disease and many other diseases. Physical inactivity can weaken your heart, muscles, and bones, lowering your metabolism and immune system. Physical inactivity can also raise your blood pressure, cholesterol, and blood sugar levels, cause weight gain, and cause mental stress. Physical inactivity can also affect the wound's healing and the valve's function after heart valve surgery.

- **Stress.** Stress, also called psychological stress, is a feeling or reaction that occurs when you face a challenge or a threat. Stress can affect your health in many ways and increase your risk of heart disease and many other diseases. Stress can trigger your body's fight-or-flight response, raising your blood pressure, heart rate, and blood sugar levels and releasing hormones, such as adrenaline and cortisol, that can damage your heart and blood vessels. Stress can also affect your mood, behavior, and well-being and cause anxiety, depression, anger, or sadness. Stress can also affect your lifestyle choices, such as smoking, drinking, eating, or sleeping. Stress can also affect the wound's healing and function after heart valve surgery.

Measure and monitor your heart disease risk factors.

To manage your heart disease risk factors, you need to measure and monitor them regularly, with the help of your doctor and health care team. You can use various methods and tools to measure and monitor your heart disease risk factors, such as:

- **Blood pressure monitor.** A blood pressure monitor is a device that measures the force of blood against the walls of your arteries. You can use a blood pressure monitor at home, a pharmacy, or a clinic to check your blood pressure regularly. You should follow the blood pressure monitor instructions correctly and record your readings. You should also share your readings with your doctor and follow their advice on lowering your blood pressure if it is too high.

- **Blood test.** A blood test is a test that measures the levels of different substances in your blood, such as cholesterol, glucose, or inflammation markers. You can have a blood test at a laboratory, a clinic, or a hospital, as ordered by your doctor. You should follow the instructions on preparing for the blood test, such as fasting or avoiding certain medications. You should also review your results with your doctor and follow their advice on improving your blood levels if they are abnormal.

- **Smoking cessation program.** A smoking cessation program is a program that helps you quit smoking and stay smoke-free. You can join a smoking cessation program at a clinic, a hospital, or online, as your doctor recommends. You should follow the instructions on how to use the smoking cessation program effectively, such as setting a quit date, using nicotine replacement products, or taking medications. You should also seek support from your doctor, health care team, family, friends, or other sources, such as support groups, counselors, or online communities, to help you quit smoking and cope with withdrawal symptoms.

- **Diabetes management program.** A diabetes management program is a program that helps you control your blood sugar level and prevent or delay diabetes complications. You can join a diabetes management program at a clinic, a hospital, or online, as your doctor recommends. You should follow the instructions on how to use the diabetes management program effectively, such as checking your blood sugar level, taking your medications, following your meal plan, and exercising regularly. You should also seek support from your doctor, health care team, family, friends, or other sources, such as support groups, counselors, or online communities, to help you control your blood sugar level and cope with diabetes.

- **Weight management program.** A weight management program is a program that helps you achieve and maintain a healthy weight. You can join a weight management program at a clinic, a hospital, or online, as your doctor recommends. You should follow the instructions on how to use the weight management program effectively, such as setting a weight goal, tracking your calories, eating a balanced diet, and being physically active. You should also seek support from your doctor, health care team, family, friends, or other sources, such as support groups, counselors, or online communities, to help you achieve and maintain a healthy weight.

- **Physical activity program.** A physical activity program is a program that helps you increase your physical activity and exercise. As your doctor recommends, you can join a physical activity program at a gym, a park, or online. You should follow the instructions on using the physical activity program effectively, such as choosing an activity you enjoy, starting slowly and gradually, warming up and cooling down, and staying hydrated. You should also seek support from your doctor, healthcare team, family, friends, or other sources, such as trainers, coaches, or online communities, to help you increase your physical activity and exercise.

- **Stress management program.** A stress management program is a program that helps you cope with stress and emotions. You can join a stress management program at a clinic, a hospital, or online, as recommended by your doctor. You should follow the instructions on using the stress management program effectively, such as identifying and avoiding your stressors, practicing relaxation techniques, expressing your feelings, and seeking help when needed. You should also seek support from your doctor, health care team, family, friends, or other sources, such as support groups, counselors, or online communities, to help you cope with stress and emotions.

Actions and choices for reducing heart disease risk factors

To reduce your heart disease risk factors, you need to take action and make choices that benefit your heart and health, with the help of your doctor and health care team. You can use various methods and tools to take action and make choices, such as:

- **Medications.** Medications are the drugs that help lower your blood pressure, blood cholesterol, blood sugar, or blood clotting and prevent or treat complications. You can take medications as prescribed by your doctor and monitor your symptoms and side effects. You should not stop or change your medications without consulting your doctor. You should also inform your doctor of allergies, intolerances, or medication interactions.

- **Lifestyle changes.** Lifestyle changes are the modifications you make in your habits and behaviors, such as quitting smoking, limiting alcohol, eating healthy, being active, and managing stress. You can make lifestyle changes as your doctor and health care team advise and monitor your progress and outcomes. You should not make drastic or unrealistic changes that may harm your health or well-being. You should also seek help from your doctor, healthcare team, family, friends, or other sources, such as support groups, counselors, or online communities, to help you make and maintain lifestyle changes.

- **Education and awareness.** Education and awareness are the knowledge and understanding that help you make informed decisions and act for your health and prevention. You can educate yourself and make yourself aware by seeking information and guidance from your doctor and health care team, as well as other reliable sources, such as books, websites, or organizations, to help you learn about your heart disease risk factors and how to reduce them. You can also be aware of the signs and symptoms of complications, such as chest pain, shortness of breath, or palpitations, and seek immediate medical attention if they occur. You can also be aware of the factors that can affect your heart function and health, such as diet, lifestyle, medications, and follow-up care, and follow your doctor's instructions and recommendations.

Managing heart disease risk factors is one of the most effective ways to improve cardiovascular health and prevent complications and recurrence after heart valve surgery. Heart disease risk factors are the conditions or behaviors that increase your chance of developing or worsening heart disease. Some heart disease risk factors are modifiable, meaning you can change or control them, such as smoking, high blood pressure, or high cholesterol.

Nutrition and Exercise for Heart Health

Nutrition and exercise are two of the most critical factors for your cardiovascular health. Nutrition and exercise can help you prevent or manage heart disease, lower your risk of complications and recurrence after heart valve surgery, and improve your quality of life. Nutrition and exercise can also help you control your weight, blood pressure, cholesterol, blood sugar, and inflammation, common heart disease risk factors.

The following information will help you understand the benefits and guidelines of nutrition and exercise for heart health, describe how you can plan and prepare for nutrition and exercise for heart health, and empower you to take action and make choices that suit your needs and goals.

Benefits and guidelines of nutrition and exercise for heart health

Nutrition and exercise for heart health can have many benefits, such as:

- Strengthening your heart, muscles, and bones and improving your blood circulation, oxygen delivery, and metabolism.
- Reducing your blood pressure, blood cholesterol, blood sugar, and inflammation, and preventing or treating complications such as infection, bleeding, arrhythmia, or valve problems.
- Enhancing your mood, energy, confidence, and happiness, and reducing your stress, anxiety, depression, and boredom.
- Supporting your personal and professional development and enabling you to resume your normal activities, such as work, leisure, hobbies, and social interactions.

Nutrition and exercise for heart health can also follow some general guidelines, such as:

- Eating a balanced and varied diet that emphasizes fruits, vegetables, whole grains, lean proteins, healthy fats, and fluids and limits salt, sugar, saturated fat, and alcohol.
- Being physically active and exercising for at least 150 minutes per week, with moderate

and vigorous intensity activities, such as walking, jogging, cycling, swimming, or aerobics.

- Following a gradual and safe process for resuming your nutrition and exercise for heart health, as guided by your doctor and cardiac rehabilitation team.
- Listening to your body and stopping or resting if you feel tired, dizzy, or short of breath.

Plan and prepare for nutrition and exercise for heart health.

To enjoy the benefits and follow nutrition and exercise guidelines for heart health, you need to plan and prepare for the process with the help of your doctor and healthcare team. You can use the following steps to plan and prepare for nutrition and exercise for heart health:

- **Assess your current situation.** You can evaluate your current physical, mental, and emotional condition and identify your strengths and weaknesses, needs and challenges, and priorities and preferences. You can also review your pre-surgery nutrition and exercise habits and determine which ones are beneficial and enjoyable to you and which ones are not.

- **Set realistic and achievable goals.** You can set short-term and long-term goals for nutrition and exercise for heart health based on your current situation and personal values and aspirations. You can make your goals specific, measurable, attainable, relevant, and time-bound and write them down or share them with someone. You can also monitor your progress and celebrate your achievements.

- **Seek help and support.** You can seek help and support from your doctor and healthcare team, as well as from your family, friends, or other sources, such as support groups, counselors, or online communities. You can ask for help or advice on how to plan and prepare for nutrition and exercise for heart health and how to cope with any difficulties or challenges. You can also give feedback and appreciation to those who help and support you.

Choices and preferences for nutrition and exercise for heart health

You are responsible for participating in your nutrition and exercise for heart health. You can choose and express preferences based on the best available information and your values and goals. Some of the choices and preferences you can make are:

- Choosing the foods and drinks you want to consume. You can choose the foods and beverages you want to consume based on your interests, tastes, and goals. You can also choose foods and drinks that are nutritious and delicious to you and avoid foods and drinks that are harmful or unpleasant to you. You can also try new foods and drinks or modify existing ones to suit your needs and preferences.
- Choosing the activities and exercises you want to perform. You can choose the activities and

exercises you want to perform based on your interests, passions, and goals. You can also choose the activities and exercises that are beneficial and enjoyable to you and avoid the activities and exercises that are harmful or stressful to you. You can also try new activities and exercises or modify existing ones to suit your needs and abilities.

- Choosing the pace and timing of your nutrition and exercise for heart health. You can choose the pace and timing of your nutrition and exercise for heart health based on your condition, progress, and comfort. You can also choose a pace and timing that are realistic and flexible and adjust them as needed. You can also respect your limits and not compare yourself to others or your pre-surgery self.

- Choosing the people you want to share your nutrition and exercise with for heart health. You can choose the people you want to share your nutrition and exercise for heart health with based on your relationships, expectations, and compatibility. You can also choose supportive and encouraging people and avoid those who are negative or demanding. You can also communicate your needs and preferences to the people you share your nutrition and exercise for heart health with and respect their needs and preferences.

Nutrition and exercise are two of the most important factors for your cardiovascular health. Nutrition and exercise can help you prevent or manage heart disease, lower your risk of complications and recurrence after heart valve surgery, and improve your quality of life. Nutrition and exercise can also help you control your weight, blood pressure, cholesterol, blood sugar, and inflammation, common heart disease risk factors.

Stress and Management Techniques

Stress management techniques are the methods and tools that help you cope with stress and emotions after heart valve surgery. Stress and emotions are the feelings and reactions that affect your mood, behavior, and well-being. You may experience stress and emotions after heart valve surgery, such as anxiety, depression, anger, or grief, as you cope with your condition, surgery, and recovery.

Stress and emotions can affect your heart function and health and increase your risk of complications and recurrence. Stress and emotions can also affect your lifestyle choices, such as smoking, drinking, eating, or sleeping. Stress and emotions can also affect the wound's healing and the valve's function after heart valve surgery.

The following information will help you understand the benefits and types of stress management techniques, describe how you can practice and apply stress management techniques, and empower you to take action and make choices that suit your needs and goals.

Benefits and types of stress management techniques

Stress management techniques can have many benefits, such as:

- Reducing your blood pressure, heart rate, and inflammation prevents or treats complications such as infection, bleeding, arrhythmia, or valve problems.

- Enhancing your mood, energy, confidence, and happiness, and reducing your stress, anxiety, depression, and boredom.
- Supporting your personal and professional development and enabling you to resume your normal activities, such as work, leisure, hobbies, and social interactions.

Stress management techniques can also be classified into two types according to how they address the source or response of stress:

- **Problem-focused   coping.** Problem-focused coping is a stress management technique that aims to change or eliminate the source of stress, such as a challenge or a threat. Problem-focused coping involves identifying and avoiding stressors, finding solutions or alternatives, setting goals and priorities, and taking actions and responsibilities. Problem-focused coping can help you regain control and confidence and reduce or prevent stress.

- **Emotion-focused coping.** Emotion-focused coping is a stress management technique that aims to change or regulate the response to stress, such as a feeling or a reaction. Emotion-focused coping can involve expressing and accepting your feelings, seeking support and comfort, practicing relaxation techniques, engaging in enjoyable activities, and reframing your perspective. Emotion-focused coping can help you calm your mind and body and cope with stress.

Actions and choices for stress management techniques

You have the right and responsibility to participate in your stress management. You can take action and make choices based on the best available information and your values and goals. Some of the actions and choices you can make are:

- Choosing the stress management techniques you want to use. You can choose the stress management techniques you want to use based on your interests, passions, and goals. You can also choose the stress management techniques that are beneficial and enjoyable to you and avoid the stress management techniques that are harmful or stressful to you. You can also try new stress management techniques or modify existing ones to suit your needs and preferences.

- Choosing the pace and timing of your stress management. You can choose the pace and timing of your stress management based on your condition, progress, and comfort. You can also choose a pace and timing that are realistic and flexible and adjust them as needed. You can also respect your limits and not compare yourself to others or your pre-surgery self.

- Choosing the people you want to share your stress management with. You can choose the people you want to share your stress management with based on your relationships, expectations, and compatibility. You can also choose supportive and encouraging people and avoid those who are negative or demanding. You can also communicate your needs and preferences to the people you share your stress management with and respect their needs and preferences as well.

Stress management techniques are the methods and tools that help you cope with stress and emotions after heart valve surgery. Stress and emotions are the feelings and reactions that affect your mood, behavior, and well-being. You may experience stress and emotions after heart valve surgery, such as anxiety, depression, anger, or grief, as you cope with your condition, surgery, and recovery.

Stress and emotions can affect your heart function and health and increase your risk of complications and recurrence. Stress and emotions can also affect your lifestyle choices, such as smoking, drinking, eating, or sleeping. Stress and emotions can also affect the wound's healing and the valve's function after heart valve surgery.

Supplements and Alternative Therapies

Supplements and alternative therapies are products and practices that are not part of standard, conventional medicine but are used to improve your health and well-being. Supplements and alternative therapies can include vitamins, minerals, herbs, dietary supplements, or complementary and alternative medicines, such as homeopathy, ayurveda, yoga, tai chi, meditation, acupuncture, or massage.

Some people with heart disease or after heart valve surgery may use supplements and alternative therapies to prevent or manage their symptoms, lower their risk of complications and recurrence, and enhance their quality of life. Supplements and alternative therapies can have some benefits, such as:

- Providing nutrients or substances that may support your heart function and health, such as omega-3 fatty acids, coenzyme Q10, vitamin D, or magnesium.

- Reducing your blood pressure, blood cholesterol, blood sugar, or inflammation, and preventing or treating complications such as infection, bleeding, arrhythmia, or valve problems.
- Enhancing your mood, energy, confidence, and happiness, and reducing your stress, anxiety, depression, and boredom.

However, supplements and alternative therapies can also have some risks, such as:

- Interacting with your medications or other supplements and causing adverse effects, such as bleeding, clotting, or arrhythmia.
- Being contaminated, mislabeled, or fraudulent, and containing harmful ingredients, such as heavy metals, pesticides, or drugs.
- Being ineffective or having insufficient or conflicting evidence to support their claims wastes your time, money, or health.

The following information will help you understand the benefits and risks of supplements and alternative therapies, describe how you can evaluate and use supplements and alternative therapies safely and effectively, and empower you to take action and make choices that suit your needs and goals.

Benefits and risks of supplements and alternative therapies

Supplements and alternative therapies can have different benefits and risks, depending on the type, dose, quality, and source of the product or practice, as well as your condition, medication, and lifestyle. Some examples of supplements and alternative therapies that may have benefits and risks for heart health are:

- **Omega-3 fatty acids.** Omega-3 fatty acids are the essential fats your body cannot make and need to get from food or supplements. Omega-3 fatty acids can help lower triglycerides, blood pressure, and inflammation and improve heart function and health. However, omega-3 fatty acids can also interact with blood thinners and increase your risk of bleeding or bruising. Omega-3 fatty acids can also cause side effects such as a fishy taste, burping, or nausea.

- **Coenzyme Q10.** Coenzyme Q10, or CoQ10, is a substance that your body makes, and you can also get it from food or supplements. CoQ10 can help your cells produce energy and protect your heart from oxidative stress and damage. However, CoQ10 can also interact with blood thinners and reduce their effectiveness. CoQ10 can cause side effects, such as headaches, dizziness, or stomach upset.

- **Vitamin D.** Vitamin D is a vitamin that your body makes when exposed to sunlight; you can also get it from food or supplements. Vitamin D can help your body absorb calcium and support bone, muscle, and immune health. However, vitamin D can also interact with calcium supplements and cause high blood calcium levels, damaging your heart and kidneys. Vitamin D can also cause side effects such as nausea, vomiting, or constipation.

- **Magnesium.** Magnesium is a mineral that your body needs for many functions, and you can get it from food or supplements. Magnesium can help regulate your heart rhythm, blood pressure, and blood sugar levels and prevent or treat complications such as arrhythmia or a valve problem. However, magnesium can also interact with some medications, such as antibiotics, diuretics, or blood pressure drugs, and affect their absorption or action. Magnesium can also cause side effects such as diarrhea, cramps, or nausea.

- **Yoga.** Yoga is a practice that involves physical poses, breathing exercises, and meditation, and you can do it at home, in a studio, or online. Yoga can help you relax your mind and body and reduce stress, anxiety, depression, and boredom. Yoga can also help you improve your flexibility, strength, and balance and lower your blood pressure and heart rate. However, yoga can also cause injuries, such as sprains, strains, or fractures, if you do not do it correctly or safely. Yoga can also be inappropriate or harmful for some people, such as those with high blood pressure, glaucoma, or osteoporosis.

- **Tai chi.** Tai chi is a practice that involves slow and gentle movements, breathing exercises, and meditation, and you can do it at home, at a park, or online. Tai chi can help you relax your mind and body and reduce your stress, anxiety, depression, and boredom. Tai chi can also help you improve your flexibility, strength, and balance and lower your blood pressure and heart rate. However, tai chi can also cause injuries, such as sprains, strains, or fractures, if you do not do it correctly or safely. Tai chi can also be inappropriate or harmful for some people, such as those with balance problems, joint pain, or heart conditions.

- **Acupuncture.** Acupuncture is a practice that involves inserting thin needles into specific points on your body, which you can do at a clinic or hospital. Acupuncture can help relieve pain, inflammation, and stress and improve your blood circulation and immune system. However, acupuncture can also cause infections, bleeding, or bruising if the needles are not sterile or inserted properly. Acupuncture can also be ineffective or harmful for some people, such as those with bleeding disorders, pacemakers, or infections.

Evaluate and use supplements and alternative therapies safely and effectively.

To evaluate and use supplements and alternative therapies safely and effectively, consult your doctor and healthcare team before starting or stopping any product or practice and follow their advice and instructions. You can also use the following tips to evaluate and use supplements and alternative therapies safely and effectively:

- **Do your research.** You can research the supplements and alternative therapies you are interested in and look for reliable and unbiased sources of information, such as books, websites, or organizations, that provide scientific evidence, reviews, or ratings. You can also compare the benefits and risks, the costs and availability, and the quality and safety of the products or practices and choose the ones that suit your needs and goals.

- **Choosing the pace and timing of your stress management.** You can choose the pace and timing of your stress management based on your condition, progress, and comfort. You can also choose a pace and timing that are realistic and flexible and adjust them as needed. You can also respect your limits and not compare yourself to others or your pre-surgery self.

- **Choosing the people you want to share your stress management with.** You can choose the people you want to share your stress management with based on your relationships, expectations, and compatibility. You can also choose supportive and encouraging people and avoid those who are negative or demanding. You can also communicate your needs and preferences to the people you share your stress management with and respect their needs and preferences as well.

Supplements and alternative therapies are products and practices that are not part of standard, conventional medicine but are used to improve your health and well-being.

Some people with heart disease or after heart valve surgery may use supplements and alternative therapies to prevent or manage their symptoms, lower their risk of complications and recurrence, and enhance their quality of life. Supplements and alternative therapies can have some benefits, such as:

- Providing nutrients or substances that may support your heart function and health, such as omega-3 fatty acids, coenzyme Q10, vitamin D, or magnesium.
- Reducing your blood pressure, blood cholesterol, blood sugar, or inflammation, and preventing or treating complications such

as infection, bleeding, arrhythmia, or valve problems.

- Enhancing your mood, energy, confidence, and happiness, and reducing your stress, anxiety, depression, and boredom.

However, supplements and alternative therapies can also have some risks, such as:

- Interacting with your medications or other supplements and causing adverse effects, such as bleeding, clotting, or arrhythmia.
- Being contaminated, mislabeled, or fraudulent, and containing harmful ingredients, such as heavy metals, pesticides, or drugs.
- Being ineffective or having insufficient or conflicting evidence to support their claims wastes your time, money, or health.

To evaluate and use supplements and alternative therapies safely and effectively, consult your doctor and healthcare team before starting or stopping any product or practice and follow their advice and instructions. You can also use the following tips to evaluate and use supplements and alternative therapies safely and effectively:

- **Do your research.** You can research the supplements and alternative therapies you are interested in and look for reliable and unbiased sources of information, such as books, websites, or organizations, that provide scientific evidence, reviews, or ratings. You can also compare the benefits and risks, the costs and availability, and the quality and safety of the products or practices and choose the ones that suit your needs and goals.

- **Start low and go slow.** You can start with a low dose or frequency of the supplement or alternative therapy and gradually increase it as needed and tolerated. You can also monitor your response and side effects and stop or adjust the supplement or alternative therapy if you experience any problems or discomfort. You can also inform your doctor and health care team of any changes or issues with the supplement or alternative therapy.

- **Keep a record.** You can keep a record of the supplements and alternative therapies you use and include the name, dose, frequency, duration, reason, and effect of each product or practice. You can also share your record with your doctor and healthcare team and update them regularly. You can also review your record periodically and evaluate the benefits and risks of the supplements and alternative therapies you use.

Supplements and alternative therapies are products and practices that are not part of standard, conventional medicine but are used to improve your health and well-being. Supplements and alternative therapies can have some benefits and risks, depending on the type, dose, quality, and source of the product or practice, as well as your condition, medication, and lifestyle.

Chapter 6

Living Well with Heart Valve Disease

Setting Goals and Milestones

After going through diagnosis, treatment, and recovery for a heart valve condition, you now enter the long-term phase of living with your repaired or replaced valve. This will require adjusting your outlook, priorities, and lifestyle to support your valve and maintain your health.

Committing to self-care and a positive attitude, you can thrive and enjoy life fully, even with a heart valve condition. Here are tips for setting and achieving goals, celebrating milestones, and finding new meaning moving forward.

- **Set both small and big goals.**

  After treatment, it's normal to feel discouraged that you can't immediately return to your regular activity levels. Setting small, manageable, short-term goals gives you a sense of progress and motivation. Aim to walk 5 minutes daily, then increase by 5 minutes weekly. Or commit to taking the stairs once this week and twice next week. Give yourself credit for each accomplishment before setting another mini-goal.

  Having larger, longer-term goals also helps provide direction and hope. Dream big, whether playing nine holes of golf, going on a memorable trip, attending a family wedding, or returning to work. Break a big goal down into smaller steps over time. Share your goals with loved ones to keep you accountable. Celebrate when you reach an important milestone.

- **Stay positive and be patient.**

  It's vital to remain patient with your limitations after valve surgery, not compare yourself to others, and focus on how far you've come. Progress will be gradual. Some days will be easier than others. Don't get discouraged by temporary setbacks. Reflect on accomplishments so far rather than what still feels out of reach. Modify goals as needed while retaining a "can-do" attitude. Listen to your doctor's guidance on safe activity timelines. With consistent effort, you will continue improving.

- **Find meaning and purpose.**
  For many, going through heart valve surgery and recovery instills a renewed sense of purpose. Use this second chance to find meaningful ways to spend time, give back, or be present with loved ones. Volunteer in your community, pick up a long-neglected hobby or learn a new skill. Rediscover activities that bring you joy and enrich your life. Share your patient experience to educate others facing similar situations. Living with intention in service of your values provides fulfillment.

- **Make self-care a priority.**

  Caring for your physical and mental health should now become a top priority. That may mean saying no to commitments that cause excessive stress or fatigue. Protect your emotional energy, limit time with negative people, and make room for uplifting relationships. Keep up with medications, exercise, nutritious meals, and doctor's visits. Listen to your mind and body. Don't neglect your needs when caring for others. Take time to recharge through relaxing activities. Managing your health and well-being lets you live well with heart valve disease.

Though you'll make some concessions, a heart valve condition does not preclude you from living a happy, purposeful life. Keep perspective, focus on what you can do versus what you cannot manage limitations constructively, and remain hopeful and forward-looking. With concerted self-care, perseverance, and a positive mindset, you can continue thriving in this next phase of your journey.

Travel and Leisure Considerations

After heart valve surgery, one of the biggest questions is when you can resume your favorite hobbies, travel, and other leisure activities. While your doctor will provide guidelines on appropriate timing and precautions for specific activities, you can enjoy much of your normal lifestyle with some adjustments. Listen to your body, gradually ease into higher-exertion activities, and use common sense to travel smartly.

- **In-town excursions and day trips.**
  Before venturing further, test out short errands, visit with friends, and go sightseeing in your city first. Start with a couple of hours away from home, then gradually increase the duration. Carry emergency contact cards and medication or medical details. Use scarves, hats, or sunscreen to protect incisions from sun exposure. Plan outings during less crowded times and allow ample time for rest periods. Enjoy local parks, museums, restaurants, shopping, and attractions as you rebuild stamina.

- **Exercise and recreational sports.**

  Returning to exercise and recreational sports you enjoy promotes immense mental and physical well-being. Start slowly under your doctor's guidance. Walking, swimming, yoga, cycling, golf, and hiking are ideal low-impact activities after surgery. Wait at least two months before introducing higher-intensity exercise involving weights, plyometrics, or heavy cardio. Listen to your body, and stop if you feel pain or dizziness. Stay well hydrated and wear sun protection. Modify sports by taking breaks, decreasing time or intensity, or choosing less strenuous versions.

- **Air travel.**

  Most patients can resume air travel 3–4 weeks after heart valve surgery unless otherwise advised by their surgeon. Request wheelchair assistance through the airport if needed. Avoid lifting heavy bags; use compact luggage with wheels. Wear compression socks to prevent leg swelling, and get up to stretch periodically on long flights. Stay hydrated.

Notify TSA agents discreetly of your surgery and carry documentation about implanted devices. Schedule a checkup after travel to ensure you tolerated it well.

- **Camping, boating, and beach trips.**
  Nature getaways are wonderful stress relievers but require some preparation. Prioritize restful destinations over action-packed ones. Use camper cabins or RVs to avoid tent discomfort. Select cabins near restrooms to limit walks at night. Pack foods that don't require extensive work to prep or cook. At beaches and pools, stay hydrated and use shade and sun protection. Wait six weeks before boating to avoid the risk of bacterial infection. Wear life jackets while onboard. Listen to your body's limits and take breaks as needed.

With your doctor's input, you can thoughtfully resume treasured travel and leisure activities that enrich your life. The key is to ease back into these gradually, take preventative measures, pack any medical supplies, and remain flexible if you need to modify plans based on your feelings. Patience, preparation, and caution will enable you to explore the world again.

Long-Term Outlook

Once you've recovered from heart valve surgery, you'll shift your focus to the long road ahead of living with your repaired or replaced valve. While incorporating some lifestyle changes, most patients can enjoy enhanced quality of life and longevity compared to before surgery. However, valve and heart issues may still arise years later. Maintaining follow-up care, managing health factors, and reporting concerning symptoms is key to your long-term outlook.

- **The lifespan of repaired or replacement valves.**
  Biological valves from animal tissue or your pulmonary valve typically last 10–20 years before needing replacement. Mechanical valves from durable polymers or metals can often last a lifetime unless blood clots develop. Talk to your cardiologist about your

specific valve's expected lifespan. Some patients may outlive their valves and require additional replacement surgery later in life.

- **Ongoing follow-up care.**
  Expect to see your cardiologist annually for the rest of your life. You may need appointments as frequently as every 3–6 months initially. Routine visits involve a physical exam, listening to your valve, EKG, bloodwork, and sometimes imaging tests. Report any concerning symptoms right away between visits. Some patients require long-term antibiotics before dental work to prevent infection. Remain diligent with medications and lifestyle modifications.

- **Potential long-term complications.**
  Even a successfully replaced valve can develop issues years later, like blood clots, leaks around the valve, stenosis, valve thickening or calcification from scar tissue, infections, and arrhythmias. Rarely, a new problem with other heart valves can also emerge over time. Your risk rises if you

smoke, are obese, have diabetes or high blood pressure, or don't take blood thinners as directed. Report any sudden symptoms to your doctor. Additional procedures may be required.

- **Emotional impact.**
  Some anxiety about the future is normal after valve surgery. Recognize when worry becomes excessive and seek counseling. Focus only on what you can control—lifestyle habits and close monitoring. Maintain regular social interaction, fulfilling hobbies, and a sense of purpose. Get educated about your heart health. Be vigilant yet optimistic, and live each day to the fullest. Your outlook impacts your quality of life as much as your physical health.

With adherence to your doctor's recommendations, you can expect to enjoy longevity along with enhanced energy and well-being for decades after valve surgery. While risks remain, valve design and surgical technique improvements offer excellent long-term results.

Conclusion

If you've made it to this final chapter, you now have a thorough understanding of heart valve disease, from anatomy and function to diagnosis, treatment options, recovery, and long-term lifestyle changes. With this knowledge, you can tackle your valve disease head-on as an informed, empowered patient.

We've covered a great deal of information across multiple complex topics. So, let's recap the key points:

1. Heart valves are crucial in regulating blood flow and preventing backflow. Damaged valves that become too tight (stenotic) or loose (regurgitant) disrupt normal cardiovascular function.

2. Valve diseases have a wide range of underlying causes, from congenital

disabilities present at birth to age-related wear and tear. Symptoms like shortness of breath, fatigue, dizziness, and swelling arise when valves lose their sealing capability.

3. Several tests help diagnose valve problems, pinpoint severity levels, and determine appropriate treatments. These include an echocardiogram, cardiac catheterization, CT scan, and MRI.

4. Medications can temporarily alleviate symptoms while exploring more permanent valve repair or replacement options. Surgery remains the gold standard treatment, but less invasive transcatheter procedures are viable alternatives for some patients.

5. Open communication with your cardiac surgeon is key to selecting the ideal valve intervention based on age, anatomy, comorbidities, and lifestyle. Recovery time and considerations vary by procedure.

6. Post-treatment focuses on cardiac rehab, nutrition, exercise, medication adherence, regular check-ups, and modifying risk factors to support your new valve and maintain heart

health. Be patient with your progress and limitations.

7. Anxiety, depression, and other emotional challenges are common after valve surgery. Seek professional counseling if needed. Draw on your support system, focus on achievable goals, and retain positivity to aid healing.

While a valve condition presents unavoidable life changes, it does not have to diminish your quality of life if properly treated drastically. Have faith in your care team, believe in your recovery, and trust your ability to adapt. Be kind to yourself on difficult days. This, too, shall pass.

Cherish the renewed energy and stamina you gain. As your strength returns, slowly revive your favorite activities, whether gardening, golfing, spending time with family, or traveling. Pat yourself on the back for the progress made while still pursuing new milestones. Share your experiences to educate and inspire other patients.

Your valve disease journey has equipped you with perseverance, resilience, empathy, and a new perspective. Allow this experience to open your mind and heart in ways you'd never imagined. Find meaning in having navigated this challenge. Let it guide you to reflect, heal, appreciate life, and live it more fully.

You now have all the tools needed to maintain optimal heart health and function for years. I wish you the best as you embark on your next chapter, and I am grateful for each new heartbeat.

Appendix

The appendix contains additional information and resources that may be useful for you to learn more about heart valve surgery and cardiovascular health. The appendix includes:

- A list of common abbreviations and acronyms used in this book and their meanings.
- A list of common medical terms and definitions related to heart valve surgery and cardiovascular health.
- A list of online sources and links where you can find more information and support on heart valve surgery and cardiovascular health.

Glossary

The glossary contains the definitions of key terms and concepts used in this book. The glossary includes:

- **Heart valve surgery:** A surgical procedure that repairs or replaces one or more of the four valves in your heart, which are the mitral, aortic, tricuspid, and pulmonary valves. Heart valve surgery can improve your heart function and blood flow and prevent or treat complications like heart failure, stroke, or infection.

- **Cardiovascular health:** The state of your heart and blood vessels and how well they function and deliver oxygen and nutrients to your body. Cardiovascular health can be affected by many factors, such as age, gender, genetics, lifestyle, and medical conditions. Cardiovascular health can also affect your overall health and well-being and your risk of developing or worsening heart disease and other diseases.

- **Heart disease:** A general term that refers to any condition that affects your heart and blood vessels and reduces your ability to function properly. Heart disease can include coronary artery disease, heart valve disease, heart rhythm disorders, heart failure, and congenital heart defects. Heart disease can cause chest pain, shortness of breath, palpitations, or fatigue. Heart disease can also increase your risk of complications, such as heart attack, stroke, or death.

- **Heart disease risk factors:** The conditions or behaviors that increase your chance of developing or worsening heart disease. Some heart disease risk factors are modifiable, meaning you can change or control them, such as smoking, high blood pressure, or high cholesterol. Some heart disease risk factors are non-modifiable, meaning you cannot change or control them, such as age, gender, or family history.

- **Nutrition and exercise:** These are the factors that involve the food and drinks you consume and the physical activity and exercise you perform to maintain or improve your health and well-being. Nutrition and exercise can affect your cardiovascular health and your risk of complications and recurrence after heart valve surgery. Nutrition and exercise can also help you control your weight, blood pressure, cholesterol, blood sugar, and inflammation, which are common heart disease risk factors.

- **Stress management:** The methods and tools that help you cope with stress and emotions after heart valve surgery. Stress and emotions are the feelings and reactions that affect your mood, behavior, and well-being. You may experience stress and emotions after heart valve surgery, such as anxiety, depression, anger, or grief, as you cope with your condition, surgery, and recovery. Stress and emotions can affect your heart function, health, and risk of complications and recurrence. Stress and emotions can also affect your lifestyle choices, such as smoking, drinking, eating, or sleeping.

- **Supplements and alternative therapies:**
These are the products and practices that are
not part of standard, conventional medicine
but are used to improve your health and
well-being. Supplements and alternative
therapies can include vitamins, minerals,
herbs, dietary supplements, or
complementary and alternative medicines,
such as homeopathy, ayurveda, yoga, tai chi,
meditation, acupuncture, or massage. Some
people with heart disease or after heart valve
surgery may use supplements and alternative
therapies to prevent or manage their
symptoms, lower their risk of complications
and recurrence, and enhance their quality of
life. Supplements and alternative therapies
can have some benefits and risks, depending
on the type, dose, quality, and source of the
product or practice, as well as your condition,
medication, and lifestyle.

References

The references contain the sources of information and evidence used to support this book's content and claims. The references include:

1. American Heart Association. (2020). Heart Valve Surgery Recovery and Follow-Up. Retrieved from https://www.heart.org/en/health-topics/heart-valve-problems-and-disease/recovery-and-healthy-living-goals-for-heart-valve-patients/heart-valve-surgery-recovery-and-follow-up

2. Mayo Clinic. (2019). Heart valve surgery. Retrieved from https://www.mayoclinic.org/tests-procedures/heart-valve-surgery/about/pac-20385276

3. Centers for Disease Control and Prevention. (2020). Heart Disease. Retrieved from https://www.cdc.gov/heartdisease/index.htm

4. National Heart, Lung, and Blood Institute. (2020). Heart Disease. Retrieved from https://www.nhlbi.nih.gov/health-topics/heart-disease

5. American Heart Association. (2020). Prevention and Treatment of High Blood Pressure. Retrieved from https://www.heart.org/en/health-topics/high -blood-pressure/changes-you-can-make-to-m anage-high-blood-pressure

6. American Heart Association. (2020). Nutrition Basics. Retrieved from https://www.heart.org/en/healthy-living/hea lthy-eating/eat-smart/nutrition-basics

7. American Heart Association. (2020). Stress and Heart Health. Retrieved from https://www.heart.org/en/healthy-living/hea lthy-lifestyle/stress-management/stress-and- heart-health

8. Mayo Clinic. (2019). Alternative medicine. Retrieved from https://www.mayoclinic.org/healthy-lifestyle /consumer-health/in-depth/alternative-medi cine/art-20046087